Library of Congress Catalog Card Number 2008929310

Printed in the United States of America

H2 WATER 4 LIFE is not intended as medical advice. It is written solely for informational and educational purposes. Please consult a licensed doctor or health-care professional should the need for one be indicated. Because there is always some risk involved, the authors and publisher are not responsible for any adverse effects or consequences resulting from the use of any of the suggestions, preparations or methods described in this book. The publisher does not advocate the use of any diet or health program, but believes the information presented in this book should be made available to the public. Any celebrity images, references, quotations, company names, organization names, or logos may not be endorsements of any specific product, service, company or their opinion. Many quotations are included throughout this book as references of what others wrote, said, or personally experienced to assist each reader in evaluating the potential of Hydrogen Water Therapy.

Published by Walk the Talk Productions
(760) 902 3343

Cover design by: https://biorave.deviantart.com

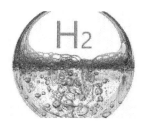

Acknowledgements

"First and foremost, I would like to thank a 'power greater than myself,' for giving me the strength, knowledge, ability and patience to undertake co-authoring 'H2 WATER 4 LIFE.' I am grateful to have persevered and completed the book satisfactory. Without this 'power greater than myself,' this would not have been possible."

Howard Peiper N.D.

"I sincerely thank the One who I dedicated my life to in 1971. You have been my Rock and source of power, justice, wisdom and the greatest love a man could ever receive."

"And, I thank every person, group, club, charity or organization mentioned below, or that is not listed below because they requested anonymity. Some of you are (or were) pioneers laboring for decades in our fields of biochemistry, alternative health therapy, naturopathic medicine and holistic healing. I am deeply humbled and grateful for everyone's many inspirations & contributions to our latest book."

Dr. Bernard Jensen, D.C. (1988), Fred Van Liew, Dr. Paul Yanick, PhD, ND, CNC, Dr. Monte Elgarten MD, Dr. Michael Kwiker, D.O. (Health Associates Medical Group – Sacramento), Julie Zones, Michele Steffney, Jim Roberts, Tyler LeBaron (MHF/MHI), Dr. Shigeo Ohta, Phd (Japan), Dr. Jan Slezak, MD, PhD, D.Sc, (Czech Republic), Dr. Jiangang Long, PhD, (China), Dr. Kyu-Jae Lee, M.D., PhD, (Korea) Dr. Mami Noda, PhD, (Japan), Joe Boccuti, David Lewis, Dr. Howard Peiper, Meg Cassell, Cindy Green (Rio Vista Beacon), Rio Vista Mayor Ron Kott, Rio Vista City Council, Jim Wheeler, Kaelee Schoennaman, D. W. Chitwood, Amanda Jenni (Center for the Arts - Rio Vista), Rev. Kathryn Morrow and Rev. Al La Far, Frank Clark, Mandy Elder (Rio Vista), B. Rhoda, Steve Ramella (Rio Vista), Jerry Robin, Toban, Emma Jones (Rio Vista), Marlene Cervantes, Sue Bielen (Rio Vista), Craig Petersen, Denise Commer (Rio Vista), LaDonna Kerton (Rio Vista), Z. Rhoda, Holly Hanes (Rio Vista).

Steven Clarke

Important Introductory Quotes

"It's an interesting parallel ... that such a <u>small</u>, indeed the SMALLEST molecule, can have a very <u>large</u> impact on human health." – Stated during a 2016 video interview by **T. LeBaron,** Founder of Molecular Hydrogen Foundation (MHF) & Molecular Hydrogen Institute (MHI) when referring to the hydrogen molecule known as molecular hydrogen and abbreviated as H2.

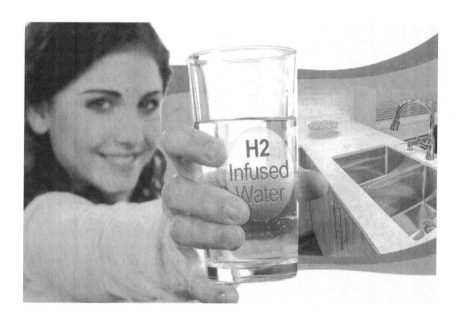

Over 1,000 Peer-Reviewed *"Scientific studies suggest H_2 has therapeutic potential in <u>170 disease models,</u> and in essentially **every organ of the human body.**"* – Molecular Hydrogen Institute (MHI) – June, 2018.

Preface

Humans have survived for as many as 90 days without food. But we can live only seventy-two hours without water before going into a semi-comatose state. However, drinking water saturated with inorganic minerals such as magnesium carbonate, calcium carbonate and other elements our bodies cannot use, may lead to a variety of unhealthy conditions and diseases. These inorganic minerals, toxic chemicals, fluoride and other contaminants can pollute, clog up and even turn our tissues into stone, causing pain, illness and even premature death. H2 Water, nature's healing water, may help remove inorganic mineral deposits and toxins from our joints, may remove cholesterol and fat, and create a pH balance in our body. This book unlocks the mysteries of H2 Water, which can often relieve chronic suffering. Using the miracle of H2 Water Therapy can now help us live healthier, happier and longer lives. - **Dr. Howard Peiper, N.D.**

We are very fortunate to be alive during a global movement towards hydrogen water therapy and enjoy its abundance of health benefits. Hydrogen was present at the dawn of time. It is the father of all known elements in our universe. It is the most abundant gas in our galaxy. Earth could not sustain life without it because 71% of our planet's surface is covered in water (2 Hydrogen Atoms + 1 Oxygen Atom = H2O). Our human body is a "bag of H2O." For centuries, science-minded people have focused on the "O" part of

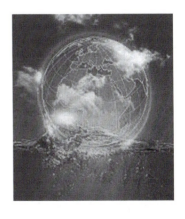

H2O and either minimized or have never considered possible health benefits of the "H2" in H2O. There are millions of hydrogen atoms in every glass of water! This raises two fascinating questions. First, how can the 2 hydrogen atoms connected to the 1 oxygen atom in H2O be separated from the water molecules? Second, how can we get these millions of liberated single hydrogen atoms to pair with each other and form a very safe, emerging medical gas, H2, … and, again, get this medical gas safely infused into a glass of water? So, in this book, we have the privilege of introducing you to what may be the greatest discovery in medical-science and health-care since 1953! - **Steven Clarke, C.M.H.A.**

Molecular Hydrogen Institute

MHI is a science-based non-profit dedicated to advancing the education, research and awareness of hydrogen as a therapeutic medical gas.

MHI collaborates with universities and institutions world-wide to advance all forms of H_2 research, in part, to establish this NexGen discovery as a very safe medical gas therapy for diseases, athletics (athletes) or other conditions in terms of prevention or treatment.

www.molecularhydrogeninstitute.org

MHI is the *epicenter* of hydrogen education and training. We encourage all to visit the MHI website to learn more, get involved, take online courses for certification, attend conferences and support MHI by voluntary work or financial donations to accelerate this exciting Global Movement.

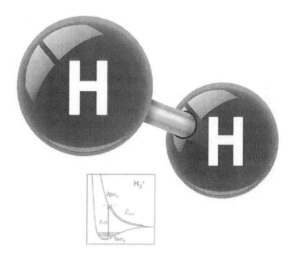

Table of Contents

"Water is the only drink for a wise man." – Henry David Thoreau

Chapter One

Welcome to Hydrogen Water 4 Life!

We warmly welcome all readers from around our globe. In the world of modern medicine, scientific discoveries and innovation drive rapid changes. We either adapt to changes, or we get left behind in old, perhaps out-of-date, even high-risk approaches to health-care. Many global doctors and researchers believe hydrogen water therapy to be one of the greatest discoveries for medical applications in 65 years. So, here and now, we declare Molecular Hydrogen as the *"Greatest Discovery in Medical-Science & Health-Care since 1953!"*

What great discovery was confirmed in 1953? The DNA molecular structure was identified and mapped out by 2 scientists who were awarded the Nobel Prize. It was composed of 2 helical chains bound to each other by *hydrogen* bonds. Medical-science was forever changed! DNA introduced us to the sub-cellular world of nano technology, epigenetics and personalized medicine.

Fast forward to 2005. Dr. Shigeo Ohta, PhD makes a huge discovery. He states: *"I was amazed at the great protective effects of Hydrogen [Gas] against oxidative stress and decided to devote my life to hydrogen medicine."* Today, in 2018, it is a global movement!

What is Molecular Hydrogen ... in Simple Terms?

H2 is two hydrogen atoms bonded together to form the **lightest** and **smallest** molecule of gas in our known universe! When infused into purified water, it produces a liquid that can hydrate virtually all 37.2 trillion of our cells at a nano or epigenetic level at speeds that are shockingly fast when seen under a microscope.

However, therapeutic molecular hydrogen gas (H2) is not new to our planet. "Healing Springs" have been around for thousands of years. The chronically ill travel to these springs (France, Mexico, India, Germany, Japan, etc.) to bathe and drink these waters. People often feel better and ailments disappear! But only recently did research confirm these waters contain dissolved hydrogen gas. Since 2007, the biochemistry and medical-science communities have exploded with over 1,000 research studies, papers, and/or some clinical studies to embrace this marvelous molecule for super-health!

How It Works

H2 is an emerging medical gas therapy with unlimited potential to restore homeostasis to essentially every organ of our body. Dixon and colleagues at Loma-Linda University report H2 has potential to help with the top 8 out of 10 disease-causing fatalities in the U.S. So, with over 1,000 documented gene expressions, how does H2 work?

- H2 alters cell signaling, cell metabolism and gene expression, giving H2 anti-inflammatory, anti-allergic, anti-obesity & anti-apoptotic (anti-cell death) effects
- H2 rapidly penetrates membranes to diffuse into our subcellular compartments, … decreasing cytotoxic oxygen radicals, protecting our DNA, RNA and proteins from oxidative stress
- H2 triggers activation or upregulation of additional antioxidant enzymes throughout our body
- H2 increases blood circulation providing hundreds of benefits

What Are Some Other Benefits of H2 Gas?

One benefit is H2 is very safe. Hundreds of studies prove its high safety profile. H2 gas has been safely used for deep sea diving since the 1940s. Hydrogen is very natural to our body, already present in our DNA and colon. And, H2 is a non-radical, non-reactive, non-polar neutral gas with no noxious side-effects!

Another benefit is its science-based anti-aging properties. Please notice this quote from a global institute of medical experts: *"The more research that accumulates about [H2], the more it appears to have the ... properties of the Fountain of Youth."* (MHI, 2018).

In this welcome chapter, we merely introduce you to H2 water therapy. Before we dive deep into H2 water, a solid foundation will be laid about our bodies, pH, dehydration, some common conditions/diseases, what is attacking us and the science of filtration and water.

"Physicians think they are doing something for us by labeling what we have as a disease"- Immanuel Kant

Chapter Two

Solved, The Secret Mystery of Aging

We are programmed to get old and look old, but it does not have to be that way. Age and longevity are relative. Some people at age sixty-five look forty-five — others at sixty-five look eighty-five.

Nobody denies genes. Our parents have a lot to do with our physical and mental makeup. But we can do a great deal to improve our looks and our quality of life. Aging without quality of life is not exciting. We can make a big difference, but only if we believe that we can, and then take action.

First and most important is to know what we put in our body. **Americans are starving and dehydrating themselves to death.** Yes, we are consuming larger amounts of "food" and "water." But Americans are getting fatter and fatter, and sicker and sicker.

Here is what is happening. We are consuming tasty foods that have calories and produce energy … but lack nutrition. Did you know that many so-called "healthy" foods have ingredients and calories that produce energy but have no nutritional value? This is the beautifully packaged commercial foods that we eat. In fact, this is mostly what Americans consume and we gradually starve ourselves to death.

Empty foods as described above do not provide nutrition. Instead, they build and accumulate as poison in our body and waste in our blood. Accumulation of these toxins in our body can be the beginning of our death. Diseases and premature death are a common expression of these accumulated toxins.

11

Think, now! Disease cannot be its own cause; neither can it be its own cure — and certainly not its own prevention. Sadly, we very often cause disease ourselves. Sickness and low quality of life go hand in hand. There is no life nor vitality in antibiotics or flu shots or immunization. Life, beauty and youth are in the blood and good blood is made of good food and good water.

Good blood, vigorous health and stamina cannot come from a subsistence on white bread, doughnuts, pies, cakes, latte's and pretty packaged commercial foods sold at supermarkets. Consider all the tens of thousands of preparations including most so-called "health foods" and "healthy" cereals. Include all the "food" that has been dyed or treated chemically to have a beautiful appearance … fried, impaired and impoverished foods … pasteurized and/or dead foods.

One of the main causes of aging and disease can be found in the derangement of normal processes of cell metabolism and cell regeneration. The accumulation of toxins (from acidic foods, waters, beverages and other sources) and metabolic waste products interferes with nourishment of our cells and slows down healthy cell regeneration and healthy new cell building. When normal metabolic processes become deranged (due to nutritional deficiencies, sluggish digestion and elimination, sedentary life, overeating, acidosis, etc.), and the process of cell nourishment, replacement and rebuilding slows down, … our body starts to grow old. Its resistance to disease will diminish and various ills will start to appear. So, an early key to anti-aging is shifting our overall body pH to being slightly alkaline.

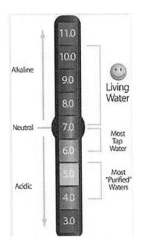

Beauty, strength, youthfulness and long life occur because we select the right foods, living waters and hydration fluids to put in our bodies. It all sounds so simple, but is it? Food is not necessarily healthy food and water is not necessarily healthy water.

"There is no natural death. All deaths from so-called natural causes are merely the end point of a progressive acid saturation." - Dr. George W. Crile

Chapter Three

Acidity - The Grim Reaper!

Accumulation of acidity in our blood, cells, tissues, organs and body fluids can be a principal factor and/or cause of disease and death. Leading researchers suggest there is no natural death. Instead, they believe deaths from "natural causes" are merely end points of a progressive acidic saturation leading to toxemia in our bloodstream.

Most of all foods we can eat are acid forming. There are so many that we cannot name them all. Almost all processed food products are acid forming. Most bottled goods, including bottled water, are acid forming. Fats, oils (modern cooking oils), sugars, sweets, syrups, candies, starches, baked goods, cereals, glucose, jams and jellies are acid forming. Nearly all cooked, fried and baked foods are acid forming.

Almost all drugs, pills, patent medicines, drinks, tonics, wine, liquors, coffee, tea, chocolate, cocoa and all manufactured foods are acid forming. Nearly all canned fruits are acid forming. All nuts are acid forming except almonds. Most peppers and pickles are acid.

The end product of our own metabolism (catabolism) is acid forming. Catabolism is our set of metabolic pathways that breaks down molecules into smaller units that are oxidized to release energy or used in other anabolic reactions. The products of combustion or oxidation in our body are acid forming. The dying leukocytes, dying tissues, the excreta in the bowels, the mucus, phlegm, dying bacteria and their toxins are all acid forming. Even brain activity, thinking, worry, temper, and all sorts of unfavorable emotions usually result in acidity. **Acidity could be called the "Father" of disease.**

When our bodies are ALKALINE, it is more difficult to get sick. When our bodies are ACIDIC, it is easier to get sick. Human alkalinity and longevity go hand in hand. Human acidity can often lead to inflammation, pain, suffering, disease, surgeries and an early funeral. However, an alkaline diet along with alkaline hydration results in better health, anti-aging and beauty.

In 2013, a scientific study and paper was published with a conclusion that acidic pH represents a novel danger signal alerting innate immunity promoting inflammation at ischemic and inflammatory sites.[1] In part, this study stated: *"Acidic extracellular pH caused rapid intracellular acidification."* In contrast, remarkably, *"alkaline extracellular pH strongly inhibited the IL-1β response to several known NLRP3 activators, demonstrating bipartite regulatory potential of pH on the activity of this inflammasome."* There is no denying this research was limited in scope to acidosis-associated pathologies, such as atherosclerosis and post-ischemic inflammatory responses. Nevertheless, its implications are biologically global to our bodies in terms of acidity being implicated in America's number one killer, heart disease!

None of us can escape wrong choices. If we live on acid-forming foods meal after meal, our body must eventually pay the bill. As acidic-forming foods accumulate, blood toxemia can gradually develop. When blood toxemia reaches a tipping point, Death (The Grim Reaper!) will often knock on our door. Therefore, acidity is a foundation of many diseases, trouble, misery, pain and tears. So, if we must eat and drink, we may just as well eat and drink healthy.

Acid in or around the nerves can result in neuralgia, neuritis, sciatica, nervousness, nerve pain, headache, earache or various nerve ailments. Acid brain matter can result in inflammation of the brain, insanity,

---

[1] Kristiina Rajamäki, Tommy Nordstrom, Katariina Nurmi, Karl E.O. Åkerman, Petrí T. Kovanen, Katariina Öörni and Kari K. Eklund. (2013) Extracellular acidosis is a novel danger signal alerting innate immunity via the NLRP3 inflammasome. *Journal of Biological Chemistry*

crime, violent passion, melancholia and hundreds of mental disease symptoms. An acidic brain cannot function normally.

Acid can cause arthritis, urinary ailments, heart valve issues and kidney problems. Acidity in or around the prostate gland can cause enlargement of the prostate, swelling and hardening, resulting in prostate cancer or, at the very least, urinary difficulties. An acidic uterus can lead to female complications of the menstrual cycle, inflammation, uterine tumors and other ailments of the generative organs.

An acidic liver may result in constipation, piles, varicosis, toxicosis, autointoxication, hepatitis, gallstones and cirrhosis of the liver.

WRONG!

Excessive acidity in our stomach can cause gastritis and heartburn. Acidity can cause gas generation and gas pressure upon our heart, diaphragm, spine and other organs. Gas pressure leads to dilation of our stomach until our stomach hangs like an empty bag, resulting in falling of our stomach, bloating, colic, indigestion, cramps and constipation. Do we see any bloated bellies in America today?

But there is hope! Many of us are waking up and taking responsibility for our own health. We are beginning to realize that, in America and in many other countries, the conventional medical and pharmaceutical establishment at the corporate level is dependent on us for its profits. This creates many conflicts of interest.

However, it is not our intention to disrespect any doctors or health-care professionals. We hold in high-regard and have very deep respect for most conventional doctors, surgeons, nurses, clinicians and other licensed health-care providers. Why? Because this global community of dedicated professionals has spent many years (even decades) saving lives by means of study, hard work and long hours in hospitals and the field!

Different diets have different effects on our health. But an acidic-dominant diet always has a harmful effect on our body. One chemical body type is subject to one kind of acidity, and another chemical body type is subject to another kind of acidity and gas formation.

So, there are many kinds of acid responses depending on the biochemistry of our unique, individual bodies. AN IMPORTANT FIRST STEP is to learn what is an acid food along with an acid water or beverage and what is an alkaline food and alkaline water or beverage. Why? Because human alkalinity and longevity go hand in hand.

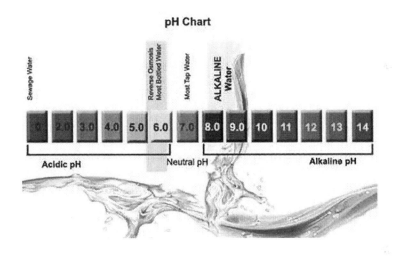

"When you are green inside, you are clean inside." - Dr. Bernard Jensen

Chapter Four

Alkalinity Conquers Death

As we grow older, it is ever more important to know the properties of food and beverages, including waters, so that we make selections that are alkaline. The very famous and highly-respected Dr. Bernard Jensen recommended a diet of 80% alkaline foods and 20% acid foods to achieve his "green inside" goal. As we live longer, there is danger of excess acid formation and gas generation. Poor elimination, low vitality, tissue acidity and autointoxication all come with age because of our ignorance of acid and alkaline foods or beverages.

Health must be developed from the inside. Beauty and youthfulness are the result of a correct alkaline diet and alkaline hydration habits. Grace in movement, elasticity in our arteries and tendons and joy in our living are all born from an alkaline bodily foundation.

When we are alkalized/balanced, there is virtually no excess acidity, no gas, no autotoxins, no poisons and no accumulation of blood toxemia. Oxygen is abundantly supplied. Our brain and nerves are well nourished and our red blood cells flow vigorously to all parts of our body. Then we can regain biological youth and enjoy a great quality of life. We can help speed up this process by drinking freshly-ionized H2 alkaline water in our daily routine.

Aging may be reversed by changing our diet and fluid intake provided we begin before we are 90 percent dead. Aging is often a disease of poor diet and dehydration. Frequently, aging can also be called a disease of progressive acid saturation. Because we are "programmed" to grow old and die does not mean that it is natural. Changing our diet and drinking ionized alkaline "H2 WATER 4 LIFE" can help slow this deterioration and, in many cases, stop this deterioration! When this occurs, we can potentially experience the anti-aging properties of Hydrogen Water Therapy!

Acid-forming foods, which should be temporarily limited during the alkalizing period, are principally meat, fish, poultry, eggs, cheese, fats, white bread, starchy foods, cakes, pastry, candy, white sugar and confections. These foods are not necessarily bad but should not be taken in quantities that exceed our body's requirement needs.

Alkaline Foods – (80% of diet)

Celery	Apples
Potatoes	Bananas
Carrots	Citrus fruits
Cabbage	Beets
Lettuce	Cucumbers
Asparagus	Melons
Tomatoes	Raisins
Green Beans	Pineapples
Squash	Grapes
Parsnips	Pears
Almonds	Buttermilk
Beans	Peaches
Spinach	Fresh Peas

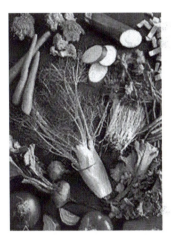

19

Acid Foods – (20% or less of diet)

Meat	Rice (white)
Fish	Corn (dried)
Poultry	Crackers
Cheese	Hydrogenated oil
Eggs	Nuts (except almonds)
Cereal	Spaghetti
Bread	White Flour
Sugar	Chocolate
Pastry	Coffee/Tea
Chips	Alcohol
Pizza	Syrup
Dried Fruit	Jam & Jelly
Candy	Cookies

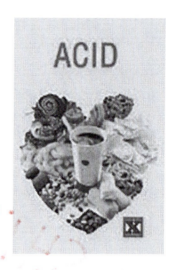

"Water is life's mater and matrix, mother and medium. There is no life without water" – Albert-Szent-Gyorgyi, Biochemist, Nobel Prize in Medicine, 1937

Chapter Five

Dehydration - Am I Thirsty?

Did you know that 50-75 percent of Americans are chronically dehydrated and many of those individuals are drinking eight glasses of water a day? Dehydration is a condition that occurs when a person loses more fluid than they take in. However, the problem is not just a lack of water, it is a lack of sub-cellular water!

Every function of the body is monitored and pegged to the efficient flow of water. "Water distribution" is the only way of making sure that an adequate amount of water along with its transported elements (hormones, chemical messengers and nutrients) reach the more vital organs first. In turn, every organ that produces a substance to be made available to the rest of the body will monitor its own rate of production. What occurs next is the release of this substance into the "flowing water," according to constantly changing quotas set by the brain. Once the water itself reaches the "drier" areas, it also exercises its many other physical and chemical regulatory actions.

Our water intake and its priority distribution are of paramount importance. The regulating neurotransmitter systems (histamine and its subordinate agents) become increasingly active during the regulation of water requirements in our body.

Water Intake and Thirst Sensations

There are basically three stages to water regulation of the body in our different phases of life. **ONE:** the stage of life of a fetus in the uterus of the mother. Interestingly, when the very first indicator for water needs of the fetus appear, the mother seems to get morning sickness during the early phase of pregnancy. **TWO:** the phase of growth to early adulthood. **THREE:** the phase of early adulthood to the demise of the person. Because of a gradually failing thirst sensation, our body becomes chronically and increasingly dehydrated, starting from the early adulthood stage. This impacts overall body pH by gradually lowering our pH until our bodies enter a state of chronic acidosis.

With increase in age, water content of the cells in our body decreases to a point that the ratio of the volume of body water inside our cells to that which is outside our cells, changes from 1.2 to 0.9. This is a drastic change. Since the "water" we drink provides our cell function and its volume requirements, the decrease in our daily water intake (less absorption) affects the efficiency of cell activity. It is the reason for loss of water volume held inside the cells of our body. As a result, chronic dehydration causes symptoms that mimic disease, especially when we don't recognize that we are dehydrated.

The human body can become dehydrated even when abundant water is readily available. We seem to lose our thirst sensation and the critical perception of needing water. Not recognizing our water need we become gradually, increasingly and chronically dehydrated with aging. Further confusion lies in the idea that when we are thirsty, many of us often substitute tea, coffee, or alcohol-containing beverages, which can act as diuretics!

A "dry mouth" is the very last sign of dehydration. Our body can suffer from dehydration even when our mouth may be fairly moist. Still worse, in the elderly, their mouth can be obviously dry and yet thirst may not be acknowledged and satisfied.

The best times to drink H2 alkaline water are: 1 or 2 glasses 20 minutes before eating any meal and the same amount two hours or more after each meal. This is the minimum amount of H2 alkaline water our body needs. If possible, 1 glass of H2 alkaline water should be taken about 20 minutes before going to bed.

Do not forget that at each phase of life, our body is the product of a series of time-operated chemical interactions. It is very possible to reverse some reactions. We need not "drown" ourselves in H2 alkaline water. The cells of our body are like sponges; it takes some time before they become better hydrated. Also, do not forget that some of them make their membranes less permissive of water diffusion, in or out.

Color of Urine

The normal color of urine should not be dark. It should ideally be almost colorless to light yellow. If it begins to become dark yellow, or even orange in color, this can be one major indicator that we are becoming dehydrated. It can mean our kidneys are working hard to get rid of toxins in our body in very concentrated urine. That is one reason why urine becomes darker in color. Dark color urine is one *negative* sign that we are dehydrated! A simple way to test urine is by using a high-quality urine test kit that offers pH test strips.

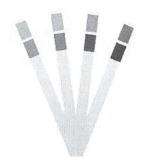

The best times to test our urine are early morning and in the afternoon. *Early in the morning,* upon awakening, establishes a baseline that we need to know. It reveals sleep activity. Most of us will test acidic. In part, this is due to our lymphatic and glymphatic systems working to drain acidic toxins and excess fluids from our bodies during deep sleep periods. *Afternoon* testing is equally important. Why? Because it reveals how H2 alkaline water progressively improves our pH. We test a minimum of 2 times. After a light lunch, we wait at least 1 hour (after a medium lunch, wait 2 hours), drink 500 ml (about 16 ounces) of alkaline water with 9 to 10 pH, wait about 20 minutes, then test. Next, we wait 20 minutes and repeat the first test (drink 500 ml) a second time. During our first 3 months, we test 3 times weekly. Thereafter, we test morning and afternoon once a week.

Later in this book, we will learn much more, in greater detail, about freshly-ionized alkaline "H2 Water 4 Life" therapy that works at our sub-cellular levels to quickly reverse dehydration and can restore our urine back to the color of a healthy newborn baby!

"The battle between life and death and humanity's struggle with sickness is over pH" – Dr. Gary Tunsky CNC

Chapter Six

pH & Cellular Health

The abbreviation pH stands for power of Hydrogen. The total pH scale ranges from one to fourteen, with seven considered neutral. Anything below seven is acidic and anything above seven is alkaline.

A healthy body functions best when it is slightly alkaline. Deviations in our blood above or below a pH range of 7.35-7.45 can signal serious symptoms of diseases. In physiology, if someone has a blood pH of 7.1 they are said to have acidosis even though, technically, 7.1 is slightly alkaline. If blood pH drops below 7.0, our body will not survive very long. When our cell and tissue pH levels deviate from a healthy range into an "acidic" state (especially below 7.0), the acidic wastes normally back up, as in a clogged sewage system.

The pH of our blood, tissues and bodily fluids affects the state of our cellular health. When our pH levels are in balance, we will experience a high degree of health and wellbeing. Every metabolic and organ/system function depends on our delicately balanced pH, including all regulatory mechanisms such as digestion, metabolism, respiration, hormone release, neurotransmitter release and immunity.

It is important to understand that pH of our blood is critical to our lives and survival. The pH of the blood has a very small degree of tolerance for variation. Our body does everything in its power to keep pH within a slightly alkaline "healthy" range, between 7.35-7.45, pulling alkaline minerals such as calcium out of our bones and other body stores, if necessary.

Blood pH Levels

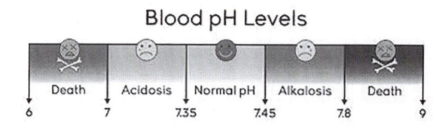

If our body is overwhelmed by excess acids from poor diet and hydration habits, or over-exposure to chemical and environmental toxins ... built-in compensating mechanisms go into effect to neutralize and excrete acidic toxins from our blood, cells, lymph and tissue fluids. There are multiple internal buffering systems our body uses to neutralize acids and balance pH. If these neutralizing mechanisms ("buffers") become overwhelmed and cannot function adequately, the excess acids will severely compromise our cellular function, eventually causing a complete metabolic and system breakdown where serious health problems such as cancer may manifest.

We live and die at the sub-cellular level. All our body's cells (37.2 trillion of them) need to be slightly alkaline and must maintain this alkalinity to function and remain healthy and alive. However, their cellular activity creates acid. This acid is what gives the cell energy and function. As each of our alkaline cells perform their task of respiration, they secrete metabolic wastes and these end products of our cellular metabolism are acid in nature.

Although these wastes are used for energy and function, they must not be allowed to build up. Most people and clinical practitioners believe the immune system is our body's first line of defense. But some medical researchers are learning that it is not. Of course, our immune system is vitally important. However, it is more like a very sophisticated clean-up service. We must instead look at pH balance maintained at a slightly alkaline level combined with H2 water therapy as our first and major line of defense against sickness and disease.

If we were to ask, "What is killing us?" … the answer might be: "acidosis." Research has shown that an acidic, anaerobic (lacking oxygen) body environment can encourage the breeding of fungus, mold, bacteria and viruses.

Calcium makes up 1.5 percent of our body weight. It is literally the human glue that holds our body together. The biggest problem scientists have found is that over time our body becomes depleted of calcium. A compound called mono-ortho-calcium phosphate is a chemical buffer for our blood. This buffer maintains alkaline level (or lack of acidity) in our blood. Without it we would die. If the pH level in our blood moves, even slightly towards acidic, we can get very sick. But to supply calcium for buffering, we must have enough calcium absorbed from our diet, waters and beverages or our body will simply extract needed calcium from our bones and teeth.

Our human body is very intelligent. It has a strategy to protect our vital organs from acidity which irritates, inflames and scars them. Fat cells can be used to store some toxins and acids from metabolic processes that are trapped in our body by lack of water. These toxins can be seen by the dark black or brown fat that comes out during liposuction. So, some (not all) toxins and acids are stored in fat cells.

When acid contacts an organ, acid can eat holes in our tissue. This may cause some cells to mutate. Oxygen levels drop in this acidic environment and calcium is depleted. As one defense mechanism, our body can make fat to protect us from our overly toxic and acidic self. Those fat cells may pack up acid and move it away from our organs. Temporarily, our fat may save our vital organs from damage. But that fat will cause so many other health problems!

Osteoporosis is very confusing for many people. Most people think they can eliminate it by increasing their consumption of milk and dairy products. But in countries where consumption of dairy products is low … the instances of osteoporosis is rare. Osteoporosis is often related to acidosis. As our body becomes more acidic, to protect against the event of heart attack, stroke, illness or even cancer, our body steals calcium from our bones, teeth and tissue. As bone mass becomes depleted, this is osteoporosis. Our body tries to protect itself with our own "stolen" calcium to bring the alkaline pH up.

One warning sign of being too acidic is an appearance of calcium deposits. Did you know there's never been a science-proven association between calcium deposits in the body and nutritional calcium? In fact, quite the opposite is found in the results of testing calcium deposits in our bodies. Calcium deposits come, not from dietary calcium, but from the structural calcium of our bones and teeth!

When our body is overwhelmed by acidosis-toxicity, mechanisms are triggered to neutralize build-up of poisonous acids to maintain a slightly alkaline pH. Alkaline solutions (pH over 7.0) tend to absorb oxygen, while acids (pH under 7.0) tend to expel oxygen. Excess acid gives our body fluids less ability to access and absorb existing oxygen. This is a spiral downward into disease. More access to existing oxygen in our body via H2 water, gives our body fluids ability to absorb more oxygen. This is an upward spiral toward health.

The first thing our body does to fight acidity is take in more oxygen the only way it knows how - through breathing harder so that it can push more CO_2 (Carbon Dioxide) out of our lungs and make room for more oxygen in our blood. We all want more energy. How many of us get winded and pant easily with a minimum of effort expended? That is low oxygen and, in some cases, an over-acidic condition plainly expressing itself when there is not enough oxygen.

In low-oxygen cellular environments, excess carbon dioxide and lactic acid collect. So, our body oxygen and intra-cellular amino acids can be used up trying to buffer these acids. Our lymph and saliva may try to neutralize and dilute the acids. However, they each thicken more as we dehydrate, thereby lowering their efficiency.

Next, our high pH electrolytes (calcium, magnesium, sodium, and potassium) are used up binding salt acids. Then our skin, urinary tract, colon and respiratory system become overloaded trying to filter them out. Next, our blood plasma changes while loading with bicarbonate to neutralize the increasing acidity. If the low oxygen and minerals and water conditions persist ... and ... there is no change in oxygen levels or diet, ... or elimination is not forthcoming, ... then our bones, teeth, muscles, joints and body fluids will be robbed of their calcium, magnesium, sodium and potassium reserves. Goodbye healthy reserves! Hello severe mineral deficiencies! Therefore, when all this fails (because acidic mucoid sludge continues to block things and pile up), ... our intelligent body can push excess acids and toxins away from its interior core of vital organs and outward to be stored in either nearby areas or in peripheral areas of our skin and extremities. Hello excess fat cells and belly fat!

Just a Few of the Hundreds of Conditions/Diseases Related to Emergency Toxin Storage

- Acid and toxins in the wrist: carpal tunnel syndrome
- Acid and toxins in the knees: osteoarthritis
- Acid and toxins in the feet and toes: gout
- Acid and toxins in the skin: dermatitis and eczema
- Acid and toxins in the joints: rheumatoid arthritis
- Acid and toxins in the tissue: fibromyalgia, chronic fatigue, and degenerative disease, etc.
- Acid and toxins in the vital organs: cancer, heart disease and serious arthritis.

The Intelligence of Sub-Cellular Health

Our genetic script runs the liver's molecular machinery to store and release sugar molecules, synthesize cholesterol, detoxify our blood, secret bile and digest hemoglobin pigment. This works in tandem with our colon cells that are simultaneously fermenting aerobic bacteria, absorbing fluid, making healthy molecular hydrogen gas in our colon and moving our breakfast through our intestinal tract.

Each of our molecules is a delicate instrument producing a flurry of electro-chemical impulses organized by ranks of molecular switches.

These turn on and off at certain intervals when necessary. A healthy body depends upon a high level of negative electromagnetic charge on our tissue cells' surfaces. Acidity generates a positive charge that dampens out these electrical fields, affecting our sub-cellular communication. Unless a treatment can remove acid toxins from our body and increase delivery of existing oxygen in our blood along with water and nutrients, ... the cure at best will only be temporary. Otherwise, the disease is driven deeper into a chronic state.

However, there is good news! If we suffer from health problems or diseases, we can abandon our past poor habits and start anew. The best and easiest way to begin treating disease symptoms or conditions is to slightly alkalize our body's pH with H2 WATER 4 LIFE, which can help dispose acids from our cells, tissues and organs.

In Chapter 15, we will explain in more detail the NexGen medical-science of H2 Water Therapy. This therapy has an unparalleled potential to revolutionize personal home health-care for hundreds of millions of families around the globe!

Before we teach you **THE SIMPLEST SOLUTION FOR OPTIMUM HEALTH**, let's continue learning about our bodies, some common conditions/diseases, what is attacking us and the science of filtration and water.

"The flow of water through cell membranes … it creates the necessary electrical energy, tops off cellular reserves, then leaves the body taking with it the waste products from each cell." – Dr. F. Batmanghelidj MD, Author & Researcher

Chapter Seven

Weight Gain, High Blood Pressure & Cholesterol

The central control system in our brain happens to recognize the low energy levels available for its functions. Our sensations of thirst or hunger also stems from low, ready to access energy levels. To mobilize energy from that which is stored in the fat we need our hormonal release mechanisms. This process takes a while longer than the urgent needs of our brain. The front of our brain either gets energy from "hydroelectricity" or from sugar in blood circulation. Its functional needs for hydroelectricity are more urgent — not only the energy formation from water, but also its transport system within the micro-stream flow system that depends on more water.

Our sensation of thirst and hunger can be generated simultaneously to indicate our brain's needs. We often do not recognize our sensation of thirst. Frequently, we assume "both indicators" (thirst and hunger) to be the urge to eat. We eat food even when our body needs to receive water. Drinking water before eating food helps to separate the two sensations. Therefore, we are enabled to eat less.

High blood pressure (essential hypertension) is one result of an adaptive process to a gross body water deficiency. When we do not drink enough water to serve all the needs of our body, some cells become dehydrated and lose some of their water to our circulation. Capillary beds in some areas will have to close so that some of the slack in capacity is adjusted for. In water shortage and body drought, up to 66 percent (66%) is lost from water held in our cells, up to 27 percent (27%) is taken from water volume held outside our cells, and about 7 percent (7%) is taken from our blood volume. Blood cells

31

then close lumen (void space just inside our cell wall) to compensate for the water loss, which in many cases, can contribute to or even cause hypertension. Therefore, one major cause for blood volume loss is a loss of body water or its undersupply through the loss of thirst sensation.

When we lose thirst sensation and drink less water than our daily requirement, some of our vascular beds will shut down to keep the rest of our blood vessels full.

When diuretics are administered to remove excess water, our body becomes even more dehydrated. A "dry mouth" from dehydration can occur and some water is taken to compensate. Diuretics cannot solve the problem of water retention because it is caused by dehydration.

Higher blood cholesterol is one sign that cells in our body have developed a defense mechanism against the osmotic force of our blood that keeps drawing water out through our cell membranes to maintain normal cell function. Cholesterol production in our cell membrane is one part of our cell survival system. It is a necessary substance. Its excess can denote dehydration.

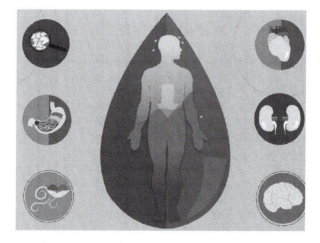

[1]www.hfhealthyliving.org A Non-Profit organization that promotes wellness through fitness, healthy food, and lifestyle guidance

In a well-hydrated cell membrane, water is the adhesive material that also diffuses through our hydrocarbon "bricks." The bilayer is separated and the space is used as a "waterway" for enzyme activity. In a dehydrated cell membrane, cholesterol is manufactured to stick our "bricks" together and prevent further loss of water from inside the cell. By drinking H2 water before eating food, we can begin to win the battle against excess cholesterol formation in our blood!

"Drinking water is like washing out your insides. Water will cleanse the system, fill you up, decrease your caloric load and improve function of all your tissues."
– Dr. Keven Stone MD, Orthopedic surgeon, researcher

Chapter Eight

Rheumatoid Arthritis & Low Back Pain

According to the U.S. Centers for Disease Control & Prevention (www.cdc.gov) updated December 27, 2017 ... *"In the United States, 23% of all adults, or over 54 million people, have arthritis. It is a leading cause of work-related disability. The annual direct medical costs are at least $81 billion."*

The U.S. CDC continues: *"The term arthritis refers to more than 100 diseases and conditions affecting the joints. The most common type of arthritis is osteoarthritis. Other forms of arthritis are gout, lupus, and rheumatoid arthritis. Symptoms of arthritis are pain, aching, stiffness, and swelling in or around the joints."*

It is estimated that about 300,000 children in the U.S. are afflicted by a form of juvenile arthritis. Once any of these conditions establishes in an individual it becomes a sentence to severe pain and suffering. So, to all of us who love our children, we shall keep reading!

Joints with rheumatoid arthritis and their pain can often be indicators of water deficiency in the affected joint cartilage surfaces. Arthritis pain can be another one of our body's regional thirst signals.

The cartilage surfaces of bones in a joint need to contain much water. The lubricating property of this "held water" is utilized in the cartilage allowing the two opposing surfaces to freely glide over one another during joint movement.

Our bone cells are immersed in calcium deposits and our cartilage cells are immersed in a matrix containing much water. As our cartilage surfaces glide over one another, some exposed cells die and peel away. New cells take their place from the growing ends that are attached to the sides of our bone surfaces. In a well-hydrated cartilage, the rate of friction damage is minimal. In a dehydrated cartilage, the rate of "abrasive" damage is increased.

Low Back Pain

According to the American Physical Therapy Association (www.apta.org) updated November 8, 2017 … *"Nearly two-thirds [2/3] of Americans experience low back pain."* This means that **over 200,000,000 U.S. Americans suffer from some form of low back pain!**

Our spinal joints, intervertebral joints and their disc structures are depended on hydraulic properties of water stored in our disc core as well as in the end plate cartilage covering flat surfaces of our spinal vertebrae. In our spinal vertebral joints, water is not only a lubricant for contact surfaces, it is held in our disc core within the intervertebral space and supports the compression weight of our upper body.

Up to seventy-five percent (75%) of the weight of our upper body is supported by water volume that is stored in our disc core which leaves about twenty-five percent (25%) supported by 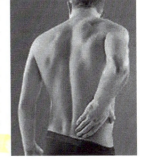 the fibrous material around our disc. A main principle in the design of all joints is for water to act as a lubricating agent as well as to bear the force produced by weight or tension produced by muscle action on the joint. Once dehydration sets in, all parts of our body begin to suffer. Our intervertebral discs and their joints are the first in line. The 5th lumbar disc is affected in ninety-six percent of cases.

"About 17 years ago, I began studying alkaline ionized water and published scientific articles on its anticancer effects ... I have now confirmed that the benefits ... are attributed to the hydrogen gas produced during electrolysis." –
Dr. Kyu-Jae Lee, M.D., PhD (South Korea)

Chapter Nine

What Happens When a Cell Becomes Cancerous?

The American Cancer Society states: *"Cancer is a complex group of diseases with many possible causes."*

According to the U.S. Mayo Clinic (www.mayoclinic.org) as of 2018, *"Cancer refers to any one of a large number of diseases characterized by the development of abnormal cells that divide uncontrollably and have the ability to infiltrate and destroy normal body tissue. Cancer often has the ability to spread throughout your body. Cancer is the second-leading cause of death in the United States."*

The Mayo Clinic continues: *"Cancer is caused by changes (mutations) to the DNA within cells. DNA inside a cell is packaged into a large number of individual genes, each of which contains a set of instructions telling the cell what functions to perform, as well as how to grow and divide. Errors in the instructions can cause the cell to stop its normal function and may allow a cell to become cancerous."*

Dr. Otto Warburg did cancer research and made a simple observation that once a cell becomes cancerous, it relies upon glycolysis for energy resulting in a higher production of acid. But he did not receive the Noble Prize for proving cancer cannot survive without oxygen or in an alkaline pH. His work shows that, under some conditions, cancer can thrive just as well in an oxygenated environment that is alkaline

36

as it does under hypoxic/anaerobic conditions. In 1931, Dr. Warburg received the noble prize for his "discovery of the nature and mode of action of the respiratory enzyme" now known as cytochrome oxidase, which transfers electrons to oxygen during aerobic metabolism.

So, what can we conclude from current research and from Dr. Warburg's research in relation to acid? First, there is no "one size fits all" approach to explaining why cells become cancerous. In other words, we cannot say that if "this condition" happens or the same "this condition" does not happen, a person's body will for certain

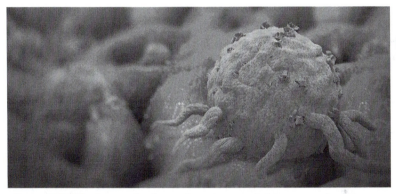

develop cancer. Second, there is a potential connection between a body remaining in an extended state of acidosis and that same body developing cancer. However, we can never say that this "connection" will always cause some of every person's body cells to become cancerous.

We cannot deny current research, accumulated over decades, points us to many causal "connections" that are either acidic, or associated with excessive acid generated and/or maintained inside us.

For example, the American Cancer Society continues: *"the known causes of cancer, [include] genetic factors; lifestyle factors such as tobacco use, diet, and physical activity; certain types of infections; and environmental exposures to different types of chemicals and radiation."* [1] Did you know that tobacco smoke is

---

[1] American Cancer Society, 2018 - www.cancer.org/cancer/cancer-causes

acidic with a 5.6 to 6.3 pH? Now, think about all that acidic smoke filling up a smoker's lungs over years or decades of smoking. Also, think about those who suffer for years from acidic "second-hand" smoke.

Research also indicates that rapid reproduction of cancer cells can use up large amounts of glucose, breaking it down into lactic acid. Lactic acid is a waste product that puts a strain on our body and causes an imbalance in our acid/alkaline ratio, or pH. As acidity of our body rises it becomes more difficult for our cells to use oxygen normally.

As cancer cells begin to multiply, forming a tumor, our liver must expend a large amount of energy converting toxic lactic acid back to glucose. The combined effect of a tumor's metabolism can be to tax our liver and acidify our body. Cancer tumors may contain as much as ten times more lactic acid than healthy tissues.[1]

Therefore, an acid condition in our body can cause our cells to become malignant. Acidity of intracellular fluids within our cells can damage each cell's nuclei which control cellular growth. Acidity in our extra cellular fluids can kill our nerve cells that connect with our brain reducing its ability to send proper messages to fight our dysfunctional cells (such as cancer cells).

But, there is hope for cancer patients! Since 2001, more scientific papers and studies have been published on the "anticancer effect" of electrolyzed (ionized during electrolysis) alkaline H2 water.[2]

---

[1] Thomas, Gordon, *Dr. Issels and His Revolutionary Cancer Treatment* (New York: Peter H. Wyden, 1973), 137-138

[2] Mr. Takaaki Komatsu, S. K., Akira Hayashida, Hirofuma Nogami, Dr. Kiichiro Teruya, Yoshinori Katakura, Kazumiti Otsubo, Shinkatsu Morisawa, Prof. Sanetaka Shirahata. (2001) Suppressive Effect of Electrolyzed-Reduced Water on the Growth of Cancer Cells. *Animal Cell Technology: From Target to Market* 1, 220-223.

Jun, Y., Teruya, K., Katakura, Y., Otsubo, K., Morisawa, S. & Shirahata, S. (2004) Suppression of Invasion of Cancer Cells and Angiogenesis by Electrolyzed Reduced Water. *In Vitro Cellular & Developmental Biology-Animal* 40, 79A-79-A.

A study in 2010 prompted Molecular Hydrogen Foundation (MHF) to state on their website an optimistic viewpoint that nine more years of research continued to support: *"Hydrogen has potential for ... suppression of cancer proliferation under some conditions."*

From Chapter 15 on, we will learn about an abundance of therapeutic properties in hydrogen water. These properties include the ability of H2 to easily diffuse into our body's sub-cellular compartments to protect DNA, RNA and proteins from oxidative stress ... and ... alter cell signaling and gene expression, giving H2 anti-apoptotic (anti-cell death) effects. This is NexGen therapy working at the nano and/or epigenetic levels to potentially protect us from cancer!

Lee, K.-J. (2004) Anticancer Effect of Alkaline Reduced Water. *J Int Soc Life Inf Sci* 22, 302-305.

Makoto Matsusuzaki, Aiko Motoishi, KuniHiko Tanaka. (2013) Mechanism of Cancer Cell Death Induced by Hydrogen. *Materials Science and Chemical Enginerring*

"One glass of water doesn't equal another. One may just appease the thirst, the other you may enjoy thoroughly. In Japan, people know about this difference"
– Heidemarie Jiline "Jil" Sander, German Designer & Writer

Chapter Ten

Did You Know There Are Only 2 Kinds of Water?

Every book needs a concise, moment of clarity chapter. This is it! Most of us would answer no to the above question. Why? Because for over 100 years, government & big business have gradually given us many choices claiming each one is both safe and healthy.

As far back as the 1910s, U.S. government agencies reassured us that the highly toxic pesticide, Chlorine, is a safe chemical we always need in our tap water. In 1945, Grand Rapids, Michigan became the first community to use a Class 4 hazardous waste, Fluoride, which spread throughout the U.S. as government agencies, again, reassured us it was both safe and beneficial at 4,000 ppb!

Next came big business. For over 40 years, a global, multi-billion dollar water industry used effective marketing tools to convince us that we can choose from an endless variety of their "healthy" waters. Think about the thousands of commercials and billboards that bombarded us with positive, happy images of their products.

It started in 1977. Perrier launched a successful advertisement campaign in the U.S., heralding a rebirth in popularity for bottled water. Today, bottled waters are the second most popular commercial beverages in North America, with about half the consumption as soft drinks. Also, in the 1970s reverse osmosis companies saw the same "liquid gold" opportunity. So, they began their marketing of smaller in-home R.O. systems to families looking for clean water. Later, pitcher and refrigerator filtered waters made their appearance.

Today, the world of water is full of choices. Right? Wrong! There are only 2 kinds of water and thus, there are only 2 choices. We can choose old, conventional, out-of-date, cheap waters that *attack* our bodies contributing or leading to over 90% of diseases … or … we can choose new, NexGen, innovative, cutting-edge, ultra-pure H2 water that can potentially *protect* our bodies from a plethora of ailments and diseases!

"Water used to be fresh, pure and drinkable. Now water has a lot of fecal matter and bacteria." – Claudine Sierra, B.S. degree in wildlife biology, researcher

Chapter Eleven

Does Well Water & Tap Water Attack Our Bodies?

Sadly, the answer to that question is an absolute yes! As of 2018, the National Toxicology Program states: *"More than 80,000 chemicals are registered for use in the United States. We do not know the effects of many of these chemicals on our health, yet we may be exposed to them while manufacturing, distributing, using, and disposing of them or when they become pollutants in our air, water, or soil."* [1]

Well Water

We must start this chapter with well water because it is the worst. Why? According to the U.S. CDC and EPA, over 15 million households obtain their drinking water from private wells which are not regulated by the EPA and not subject to their standards.

Most private wells do not have experts regularly checking the water's source before it is sent to the tap. Families that use private wells must take special precautions to ensure their drinking water is safe.

How Does Well Water Become Contaminated?

- ❖ Seepage Through Landfills
- ❖ Underground Storage Tanks
- ❖ Fertilizers & Pesticides
- ❖ Runoff from Urban Areas

---

[1] https://ntp.niehs.nih.gov/about (2018)

- ❖ Flooding from Large Amounts of Rainfall
- ❖ Decades of "Acid Rain" Seeping into Aquifers
- ❖ Failed Septic Tanks
- ❖ Mining & Factories
- ❖ Nuclear Waste Disposal Sites (39 U.S. States)

Is Well Water Really That Bad?

Yes! Marla Cone wrote in Environmental Health News: *"Private drinking water wells are ... often contaminated with potentially dangerous elements. Throughout the nation, metals and other elements are tainting water wells at concentrations that pose health concern. For one element – manganese – contamination is so widespread that water wells with excessive levels are found in all but a few states. Arsenic, too, is a national problem."* [1]

According to the CDC & EPA in 2017, the 17 most common diseases and contaminants found in well water are: Arsenic, Copper, Cryptosporidium, Campylobacter, E. Coli, Enterovirus, Gasoline, Giardia, Hepatitis A, Lead, Manganese, Nitrate, Norovirus, Radon, Rotavirus, Salmonella, and Shigella.

Tap Water

America's aging pipelines have been there a long time. Parts of the water system are over 100 years old! In many areas, water supply was originally built to supply a few thousand people. So, those aging pipes were laid for a very different America of 100 years ago. In many other countries, there are aging pipelines that are even older!

In Flint Michigan, their tap water contained high toxic levels of lead. But Flint is not alone. The water-bearing infrastructure across the U.S. is in trouble and the "cracks" are, literally, showing. Thousands of chemicals have found their way into our well waters and tap waters. Even if our water is cleaned up at a treatment plant, it is estimated that "clean" water can take a 3 to 7-day journey to our homes through a

---

[1] Marla Cone, Editor-In-Chief *Environmental Health News* (2011)

network of aging pipes that often introduce new contaminants into our water.

As of 2017, only 93 contaminants are regulated by the EPA. This leaves over 79,900 unregulated!

If we want to have safe drinking water, a first step is to understand the kinds of pollutants that may be in our well water or tap water. The following are extremely dangerous health-threatening pollutants:

- Pathogens
- Toxic minerals and metals
- Organic chemicals
- Radioactive substances
- Additives
- Disinfection-by-Products (DBPs)

Pathogens

Pathogens are harmful microorganisms such as bacteria, viruses and parasites. They can cause such diseases as typhoid, cholera, hepatitis, flu and giardiasis. The most common bacteria are closely monitored in public water supplies. Private wells may often be contaminated with bacteria. Some wells are near a septic system or open to the air and can be exposed to chemical pollution or animal fecal matter.

Viruses are smaller than bacteria and harder to detect. Viruses are common in water. A third type of pathogens found in water are protozoan parasites. In people that have a suppressed immune system, these can be life threatening.

Toxic Minerals

Toxic minerals are the harmful inorganic substances that are found in water supplies. They include metals as well as common minerals in the form of rock, sand, and clay. The toxic substances in water that are known to be harmful to our health in excessive quantities are:

Aluminum	Chromium	Nitrate
Arsenic	Copper	Selenium
Asbestos	Fluoride	Silver
Barium	Lead	Nitrite
Cadmium	Mercury	Uranium

These toxic minerals and inorganic compounds occur naturally in water, and they also enter water from man-made sources.

Organic Chemicals

Organic chemicals are substances that come directly from, or are manufactured from, plant or animal matter. Plastics, for example, are organic chemicals that are made from petroleum, which originally came from plant and animal matter. There are over 80,000 different manufactured, or synthetic, organic chemicals in commercial use today. Many of these organic chemicals have found their way into water supplies. New and dangerous ones are created in the process of water treatment. Chlorine, which is added to essentially all U.S. public supplies, combines with organic compounds from decaying plant matter or sludge found in water system pipes, to form a category of toxic pollutants called trihalomethanes (THMs) that are known carcinogens (substances that increase a risk of getting cancer).

Radioactive Substances

Radioactive substances in water fall into two categories: radioactive minerals and radioactive gases. Radioactive minerals can be either naturally occurring or man-made. Man-made sources of radioactive minerals in water include nuclear power plants, nuclear weapons facilities, radioactive material disposal sites and docks for nuclear-powered ships. Another source of radioactive pollution comes from hospitals, which dump low-level radioactive wastes into sewers. Add to this, millions of hospital patients treated each year with radiation or radioactive fluids who urinate into hospital toilets that flush millions of gallons of toxin urine into sewers. Some of those radioactive wastes eventually find their way into our water supplies.

Additives

Most public water treatment plants add things to water. These are added for a variety of reasons, ranging from disinfection to enhancing effectiveness of treatment to improving water's aesthetic qualities. The best-known additive is chlorine. However, chloramines and chlorine dioxide are also used.

•• MMS

In 2013, it was reported [1] the EPA estimates Americans are consuming 300-600 times the amount of chlorine considered safe via tap water, hot baths and hot showers (vaporizing chlorine into gas) along with swimming in pools and sitting in hot spas or jacuzzi hot tubs. Overall risk of getting cancer is 93% higher in people exposed to chlorinated water. There are 50-60% higher levels of chlorination in breast tissue of women with breast cancer than women without breast cancer. No wonder Dr. R. Carlson (Univ. of Minnesota) declared: *"Chlorine is the greatest crippler and killer of modern times!"*

Fluoride

Did you know that fluoride is a Class 4 hazardous waste material, almost as toxic arsenic? It has been added to public drinking water since the 1950s, despite evidence of its health hazards. According to research, fluoride consumption creates multiple links to cancer. Fluoride can cause cancer, transforming normal human cells into cancerous ones, even at only 1 ppm (parts per million), the official "safe" dosage set by U.S. Public Health Service for drinking water. We could write an entire book on the dangers of fluoride. For now, let's close this sub-heading with three sobering comments, the last 2 from highly-respected doctors with unimpeachable credentials:

---

[1] Alanna Ketler, The Harmful Affects Of Chlorine Published in CE Magazine www.collective-evolution.com August 15, 2013

"It appears that fluoride can cause Down's syndrome, Alzheimer's, birth defects, cancers, recurrent rashes, mouth ulcers, headaches, and osteoporosis. It also presents serious risks to diabetics and may be fatal for people suffering from kidney dysfunction." [1]

Dr. Dean Burk PhD, 34 years at U.S. National Cancer Institute, went on Congressional Record July 21, 1976: *"Fluoride causes more human cancer death and causes it faster than any other chemical."*

Dr. Albert Shatz, American Microbiologist, Co-Discoverer of antibiotic streptomycin, Nobel Prize Laureate, after studying fluoridation from 1956-2003, said: *"Fluoridation is the greatest fraud in the world against the greatest number of people."* [2]

Disinfection-by-Products (DBPs)

Today, the most common disinfection chemicals used at water treatment facilities are chlorine, chloramines, and chlorine dioxide to kill harmful, disease-causing microorganisms in the water. Scientists discovered that toxic disinfection-by-products (DBPs) form when these chemicals react with natural organic matter like decaying vegetation along with biofilms present within source water or distribution pipes.

More than one respected doctor, researcher, biochemist and chemical engineer have warned that DBPs are over 1,000 times more toxic than chlorine [3] … and so … out of all the other toxins and contaminants in tap water, DBPs appear to be the worst of the bunch. Why? Because they are very highly carcinogenic!

The top 5 DBPs are trihalomethanes (THMs), halocetic acids, bromate, chlorite and trichloramine. Chloroform is a DBP within the family of THMs. We can look for them in our city's water report.

---

[1] Peggy Sidor, www.fluoridealert.org February 2, 2001

[2] https://library.temple.edu/scrc/albert-schatz-papers (Temple University)

[3] Dr. Paul Connett PhD and Floyd Maxwell, BASc (Chemical Engineer)

Environmental Defense Fund states: *"Although concentrations of these carcinogens are low, it is precisely these low levels that cancer scientists believe are responsible for the majority of human cancers in the United States."*

Concentrations of chloroform and trichloramine both in and above swimming pools are causing asthma in regular swimmers, with indoor pools accelerating onset of or exacerbating many breathing disorders.

What About "Raw" Water or Collected Rain/Atmosphere Water?

Based on scientific research and what we have learned in this chapter, it should be clear that drinking unfiltered raw or rain water for extended periods can lead to serious health problems and diseases!

"Myths which are believed in, tend to become true." – George Orwell, Novelist

Chapter Twelve

Filtered Water – Moneymaking Marketing Myths!

So, now that we know most well waters and all tap waters are attacking our bodies, let's begin this chapter by agreeing on two points. *First,* source water coming into our homes needs to be filtered to remove hundreds of contaminants of which only 93 are regulated. *Second,* we should choose the most advanced filtration system our hard-earned money can buy. As mentioned in Chapter 10, today's billion-dollar home filtration industry got started in the 1970s. Decade by decade, a variety of water filtration systems from small to medium to whole house systems came to be offered to consumers. Each filtration device or system claimed to be "the best" at something and each company's "word wizards" developed marketing campaigns to persuade families to buy their product. Let's now examine the most common filtered waters in order of their appearances.

Reverse Osmosis (RO)

Across America, we see Reverse Osmosis (RO) filtration systems installed under kitchen sinks. This technology had its beginnings in the 1960s … but was never intended for use in residential homes!

RO water was designed for and is needed for specific applications. First, it is vital for industrial, technical and laboratory purposes. Second, it has meant that people in dire situations around the world can drink clean water. Troops and civilians in battle-torn countries or people in disaster areas who lost their infrastructure can use reverse osmosis to make clean, drinkable water.

However, is long-term drinking of RO water healthy? Absolutely no! Most people do not know that RO water is too clean. The filtering process removes contaminants; but it also removes the good things our bodies need to thrive. Essential minerals such as calcium and magnesium are completely removed, which are vital for our bones, teeth, muscles, blood vessels and heart. As a result, RO water is often referred to as "dead" water. A simple test using a TDS (Total Dissolved Solids) meter can confirm just how dead RO water is. Another problem, … RO water is usually acidic. Many people report that it does not even seem to quench their thirst!

Does RO water act like a parasite? Yes! Water has been called the universal solvent. A solvent is a substance (usually liquid) that dissolves a solute (usually a solid) into a solution. Being void of minerals, reverse osmosis water is unstable, aggressive and parasitic. It wants to stabilize itself. How? Once inside our mineral-rich bodies, it will seek out and leach minerals from our bones, teeth, muscles, tissues and other body parts.

When RO water is done taking our available minerals, this parasitic water carries them away in our urine. Goodbye minerals! If we drink RO water over an extended period, we can experience severe mineral deficiency. If we cook with RO water, it's even more shocking. Magnesium, calcium and other beneficial minerals can be reduced between 60% to 86%!

In recent years, some RO companies have claimed to address this serious problem by adding a re-mineralizing cartridge to their system just before water is delivered through its faucet. However, there are usually no specifics that RO companies include with their marketing materials disclosing the exact minerals, amounts and ratios of minerals, nor any disclosure of all the missing trace minerals no longer present in their filtered water needed as "co-factors" to insure their RO water is now healthy water. So, with no scientific studies nor any evidence to support their claims, a moneymaking marketing myth that "RO water is the purest and healthiest water" continues to persuade people they are making a great, healthy choice.

An even greater concern is that household reverse osmosis units are not bacteria proof! Many factories, located in distant places, make

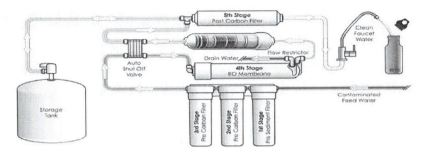

membranes that are "clean" but not certified sterile, bacteria-free. So, it is very possible that a new membrane is already contaminated with bacteria or bacteria will move up the seal that holds the membrane.

Also, mold and bacteria may grow when the RO system is not being used for some time or household temperatures increase past 80 degrees and beyond. These two conditions can impact the RO tank and other internal parts where water is stagnant.

With all these health risks associated with household reverse osmosis units, it is no surprise that Dr. Frantisek Koziek, M.D., Phd, Head of the National Reference Centre for Drinking Water in Czech Republic said: *"the exposure and risks should be considered not only at the community level, but also at the individual or family level."* [1]

Distilled

Globally, families drink and cook with distilled water. But it was never intended for use "at the individual or family level." Rather, like its "brother" RO water, distilled water was designed for specific applications. First, for chemistry, laboratory research, perfume making, some food production and in a medical environment, it is irreplaceably useful. Second, during a natural disaster when our home

---

[1] http://www.who.int/water_sanitation_health/dwq/nutrientschap12.pdf

water sources are contaminated, distilling or boiling water may be the only temporary way to get some "clean" water.

So, is distilled water healthy for drinking and cooking? No! Home distillers remove essential minerals from our water. Just like RO water, distilled water is also "dead" water.

Is distilled water acidic? Yes! Distilled water is an active absorber. When it contacts air, the oxidizing properties of carbon dioxide and oxygen making it acidic. Dr. P. Airola N.D., Phd wrote about dangers of distilled water in the 1970s when it was a fad with health food enthusiasts. He warned: *"Distilled water is totally devoid of minerals, and prolonged use may leach out the body's own mineral reserves and lead to severe mineral deficiencies and such diseases as osteoporosis, diabetes, tooth decay and heart disease."*

Even with health warnings, industry analysts predict that "distilled water will thrive even more 10 years from now."[1] Again, companies that sell in-home distillers have "word wizards" who developed marketing campaigns to persuade families to buy their products.

Pitcher (Jug-Type) & Refrigerator

Let's keep this very simple. Is drinking water filtered through these systems better than drinking tap water? Yes, of course! However, the following 2 points should be enough to steer us away from these.

First, we usually get what we pay for. We need to stop and think. How much of the "bad stuff" can these inexpensive pitcher & refrigerator filters remove? Answer: Most inexpensive filters only remove a small percentage of just some, or even a few toxins. For example, let's take arsenic, fluoride or uranium, and let's be generous and say that one of these filters can remove 10% of these poisons. That means we would still be drinking 90% of these poisons!

---

[1] http://all-about-water-filters.com/future-of-the-distilled-water-industry/

Second, remember the "word wizards" are way ahead of us via their moneymaking marketing myths. Read the vague language used in their commercials or on their packaging. We will see, hear or read "reduces" or "tastes better" or "great tasting for over 20 years!" But frequently, when a specific chemical or contaminant is mentioned, like chlorine, fluoride or lead, we will only be informed that the device "reduces" or there will be no claim at all!

TDS & Guess WHO Busts Their Myths?

The World Health Organization (WHO) was very concerned about severe health risks of new filtration methods that produce "demineralized," low Total Dissolved Solids (TDS) water. A final report, published in 1980, issued strong warnings to the world and home water filter industry, busting their marketing myths! You can read, in just 12 pages, how dangerous these waters are. Let us close this chapter with their warning: *"Demineralized [low TDS] water ... has a definite adverse influence on the animal and human organism."*

"I will REFUSE disposable plastic."
– Plastic Pollution Coalition

Chapter Thirteen

Bottled Water & Plastic Bottles

There are times when drinking bottled water is necessary. When? During emergency situations where local "clean" water sources are cut off, in short supply or contaminated. Bottled water could mean the difference between life and death for people in earthquake, flood or war-torn countries during relief periods. Or, when camping or traveling to an area with parasite-infested water or high levels of contaminants, bottled water is a good thing.

However, should we drink most bottled waters on a regular basis? Positively no! Here are three (3) of many reasons why.

Reason #1. Bottled water is often toxic! In a study by German researchers, over 24,500 chemicals were found lurking in bottled water. [1] In a U.S. study, [2] the NRDC (National Resources Defense Council) tested over 1,000 bottles and 103 brands using 3 independent labs. About one-third (1/3) of bottled waters contained significant contamination (i.e., levels of chemical or bacterial contaminants) including coliform bacteria, HPC bacteria, pseudomonas aeruginosa bacteria, arsenic, nitrate, trihalomethanes and phthalate.

Reason #2. Bottled water has little health value. To be truly healthy, water needs to have all 3 of the "A" properties. Healthy drinking water should be alive with molecular hydrogen and minerals, alkaline

---

[1] Dr. Jennifer Landa. www.foxnews.com/health/2014/01/13/more-than-24500-chemicals-found-in-bottled-water.html
[2] www.nrdc.org/sites/default/files/bottled-water-pure-drink-or-pure-hype-report.pdf

and full of antioxidants. Most bottled waters fail in one, two or all 3 of these properties. In other words, most bottled waters are "dead," acidic and/or even toxic!

Reason #3. Bottled water is expensive. Today, a gallon of bottled water is often more expensive than a gallon of gas. According to the Huffington Post, bottled water is 240 to 10,000 times more expensive than tap water. Yet, Americans still spend $15 billion annually!

What About Plastic Bottles?

First, did you know that a recent investigation by Environmental Working Group (EWG)[1] confirmed over 80 plastic contaminants can leach into water in plastic bottles? PET (or PETE) plastics, the type used to make plastic water bottles, contain dozens of chemical additives, manufacturing impurities and breakdown byproducts … more than 80 potential contaminants that can leach into water. According to research by 5GYRES, people are *"eating microplastics"* and *"98% of Americans test positive for the chemicals found in plastic."*

So, people all over the globe are usually paying for and drinking a bottle of water contaminated with toxic plastic resins, chemicals or compounds … in every plastic bottle they buy!

Second, we all know that plastic bottles are a waste disposal nightmare. According to some chemists, the average time for a plastic bottle to completely degrade is at least 450 years!

Yet, American Chemistry Council and the Association of Plastic Recyclers report a 2-year decline in recycling for plastic bottles of all resins. [2] How bad is it? U.S. plastic bottle recycling rate fell to 29.7 percent in 2016, less than 1 out of every 3 bottles!

---

[1] www.ewg.org/research/ewgs-water-week/mad-monday-what-you-dont-know-may-hurt-you#.Wun5k4gvyUk

[2] https://resource-recycling.com/recycling/2017/11/07/bottle-recycling-rate-falls-second-consecutive-year/

This huge waste disposal, ecological and personal health crisis is mobilizing groups of all sizes to reverse the trend and move our world towards safer, more sustainable water container solutions. Below are just a few non-profit organizations that can teach us about this global crisis and we can support by our personal efforts and donations.

www.5gyres.org

www. plasticpollutioncoalition.org

www.banthebottle.net

"Parents who give children energy drinks might as well be giving them cocaine." – Jamie Oliver (Evening Standard) Celebrity Chef & Author

Chapter Fourteen

Sports Drinks, Energy Drinks & Other Supplements

Sports & Energy Drinks. Most of us know these drinks are merely a short-term "fix" to a bigger problem … the need for rehydration and increased energy. So, we give in to marketing campaigns and convenience in exchange for drinks that can seriously harm our body's long-term health. Let us group these two together with just some of their dangers.

- Stimulants like Caffeine
- Sugar, high levels, from GMO corn, high fructose corn syrup
- Excessive B Vitamins
- Artificial Sweeteners (Aspartame, Sucralose & Saccharin)
- Phenylalanine (can behave as a neurotoxin) – ADD/ADHD
- Citric Acid (Preservative)
- Potassium Sorbate (Preservative)
- Sodium Benzoate, Benzoic Acid & Benzoate (Preservative)
- Colorings (Chemical dyes such as Sunset Yellow)

Hundreds of studies link excessive stimulants and sugar to heart problems and diabetes. Two studies showed potassium sorbate (PS) can mess with DNA. One more study proved PS is genotoxic to human white blood cells. Another study revealed PS mixed with ascorbic acid (Vitamin C) caused mutagenicity and DNA-damaging activity.

What about benzoic acid (BA)? When BA is combined with citric acid, the highly carcinogenic benzene is produced! Below are a few helpful resources to help us move away from these dangers.[1]

Other Supplements (Portable Mixes & Electrolyte Products)

A new category of portable mixes recently emerged called "water enhancers" designed to add flavor, sweetness and, in some products, a few healthy minerals. Some are powders and others are packaged as liquids in squeeze bags or plastic containers.

One major name brand we will call "Brand X" sells flavored enhancer drops. Notice what ingredients are included:

❖ Citric Acid
❖ Sucralose
❖ Potassium Sorbate
❖ Red 40 & Yellow 6

What is the goal of "Brand X?" Their advertisements say to 'add our drops to our clean, pure bottled water.' Their marketing is crafted to get us to buy a new product and buy more of their bottled water to increase sales and profits! But, do we remember how dangerous these ingredients can be, when combined with each other, as explained in our previous page? Many dieticians and naturopathic doctors warn against using these water enhancers. Johannah Sakimura, RD said: *"don't fall for the healthy hype"* and strongly cautioned: *"many of these drink mixes are loaded with fake, chemical additives."*[2] And what about all the electrolyte products we can now add to our water? According to Nina Anderson, SPN, most electrolyte products do not contain all the needed trace minerals for maximum rehydration and

---

[1] www.thehealthyhomeeconomist.com/sports-drinks-hide-aspartame/ 4/28/2018
Craig Elding www.thehealthcloud.co.uk/ingredients-in-sports-drinks/ 7/6/2012
http://www.bioline.org.br/pdf?pr16025 Published January, 2016
[2] Johannah Sakimura, RD https://www.everydayhealth.com/columns/johannah-sakimura-nutrition-sleuth/water-enhancers-dont-live-up-to-name/
Cocktail of Death http://seattleorganicrestaurants.com/vegan-whole-food/toxic-ingredients-in-energy-drinks.php

absorption. In addition to primary minerals (calcium, magnesium, potassium, etc.), we need *"trace amounts of selenium, boron, copper, manganese, zinc, cobalt, silica, iodine and chromium."*

Later in this book, a special chapter will help us understand the science-based reasons why most electrolyte products can fail miserably to achieve the real healthy hydration goals we all seek.

"Water is the best of all things" – PINDAR, Greek Lyrical Poet (522-438 BC)

Chapter Fifteen

What is H2 Water Therapy?

H2 is an emerging medical gas therapy with unlimited potential to restore homeostasis to virtually every organ of our body. What is homeostasis? In simple terms, it is the condition of seeking or maintaining dynamic equilibrium (balance) within a cell or our entire body. It requires constant adjustments as conditions change inside and outside our cells via complex feedback loops. Therefore, what happens at the cellular and sub-cellular level impacts all our body's systems, organs and parts. As MHI confirms: *"Hydrogen is not considered a powerful drug, and as mentioned only helps bring the cell/organ back to homeostasis without causing major perturbations."* [1]

Homeostasis Is First Key to Optimum Health!

When our overall body achieves homeostasis, we feel stable, healthy, vibrant and sometimes even younger! Why? Because each of our body systems contributes to the homeostasis of our other systems. No system in our body works alone and our well-being depends upon the well-being of all our interacting body systems. A disruption within one of our systems usually impacts other body systems. Most of these systems are controlled by hormones released from our pituitary gland. Here are 4 main examples of homeostasis inside our bodies:

- Regulates amounts of water and minerals in our body (osmoregulation). This happens primarily in the kidneys.

---

[1] www.molecularhydrogeninstitute.com/hydrogen-an-emerging-medical-gas 2018

- Removes metabolic waste (excretion). This is done by excretory organs such as our kidneys and lungs.
- Regulates blood glucose level. This is mainly done via our liver, with insulin and glucagon secreted by our pancreas.
- Regulates body temperature. This is mainly done by our skin.

Did you notice how water is involved in all 4 examples of homeostasis? Thus, any therapy we explore for therapeutic potential must demonstrate verifiable success or failure to interact with water. Why? Because water is involved in essentially every bodily function!

Water & H2 Are the Keys to Homeostasis!

Most of us assume that mostly blood is flowing through our 60,000 mile circulatory system. We are surprised to learn that only about 12% of the fluids moving through our "blood stream" are blood! The other 88% is water. Medical school textbooks vary. But nearly all of them agree on these estimates (+/-) for an average adult:

- ❖ Average percentage of water in the total body mass of a healthy adult body is about 60% (+/- for gender or age)
- ❖ Fluid distribution in our body is divided into 2 compartments. First, intracellular (ICF) has about 28 L (= 7.4 gallons); Second, extracellular (ECF) has about 14 L (= 3.7 gallons) for a total of about 42 L (= 11.1 gallons)
- ❖ Total blood volume (plasma, red blood cells, white blood cells & platelets) is about 5 L (= 1.32 gallons)
- ❖ 5 L of blood divided by 42 liters of water fluids = 11.9%

This is an "Ah-Ha!" moment for many of us. We truly are "skin bags" of water. Essentially every bodily system and organ needs water to achieve its own homeostasis. There are many estimates of the percentage of water in our body parts and organs. Here are just a few examples that are not precise since they can vary from person to person along with each person's ever-changing internal conditions. [1]

---

[1] https://water.usgs.gov/edu/propertyyou.html
Anne Marie Helmenstein Ph.D. / Chemistry Expert (Nov/2015)

Eyes 95%	Lungs 83%	Muscles & Kidneys 79%
Liver 70-75%	Brain & Heart 73%	Skin 64%
Bones 31%	Hair 10-13%	Teeth 8-10%

Now, if we combine purified, healthy water with the smallest and lightest molecule in the universe, H2, we can enjoy the simplest solution for optimum health: Hydrogen Water Therapy! Notice just a few of our bodily functions that require healthy water.

What Does Water do for You?

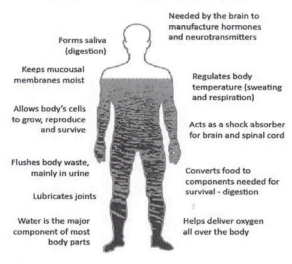

Needed by the brain to manufacture hormones and neurotransmitters

Forms saliva (digestion)

Keeps mucousal membranes moist

Regulates body temperature (sweating and respiration)

Allows body's cells to grow, reproduce and survive

Acts as a shock absorber for brain and spinal cord

Flushes body waste, mainly in urine

Lubricates joints

Converts food to components needed for survival - digestion

Water is the major component of most body parts

Helps deliver oxygen all over the body

H2 Water Therapy Has 3 Sought-After Properties

Why are so many global doctors and scientists excited about this discovery and its NexGen applications to modern medicine? Because hydrogen water therapy has 3 unique, sought-after properties.

- o Studies *"demonstrate its high safety profile."*
- o Therapeutic potential in hundreds of diseases
- o Offers a simple, universal approach to personal home health-care, … because nearly everybody already drinks water!

When compared to strong medications and chemotherapeutic agents with noxious, even toxic side effects, H2 has no noxious effects yet to be reported. H2 has potential to prevent or treat hundreds of diseases. H2 could become the "gold standard" for families to use as an alternative, naturopathic in-home therapy that is easy-to-implement.

Why All of Us Need Molecular Hydrogen Therapy

Here is a dose of reality. No matter how young, strong, or healthy we may think we are … an appearance that our body is healthy does not guarantee we are disease-free. Disease can get a foothold in our body without our awareness. How? Our overall good health and appearance of being strong and fit can mask a disease for years. Then, "suddenly" something changes in our life that weakens our immune system and pushes our entire body out of homeostasis.

Prior to this, our entire body may not have been in complete homeostasis. We just assumed it was because no loud alarms went off. However, if our body was not receiving a daily therapeutic dose of H2 water that was purified via a filtration system that is verified to remove hundreds of contaminants, it is likely we were hydrating with waters or other beverages that were either "dead," acidic and/or even toxic! Under these circumstances, disease can hide for years. Below are just some of the many conditions and diseases people suffer through or can be "suddenly" diagnosed with:

Low energy	Tumors	Autoimmune Diseases
Sleeping problems	Arthritis	Liver Disease
High blood pressure	Osteoporosis	Dementia
High Cholesterol	Weight problems	Parkinson's
Skin / Rash issues	Water retention / Edema	Kidney Disease
Acid Reflux	Kidney stones / Gout	Influenza & pneumonia
Intestinal troubles	Prostate issues	Diabetes
Irregular bowels	Migraines	Alzeimer's
Ulcers	Cataracts / Glaucoma	Strokes
Pain issues	Colitis	Respiratory Disease
Nerve disorders	Thyroid/Adrenal issues	Heart Disease
Gluten sensitivity	Celiac Disease	CANCER

All of us need molecular hydrogen therapy primarily for prevention. Why wait for a "sudden" diagnosis? We can have a NexGen personal home health-care system that proactively protects and prevents diseases from, in many cases, not even starting! However, at the same time, a NexGen naturopathic health-care system can also be reactively used for treatment. Later you will read unsolicited, verified testimonials from real people sharing how H2 water therapy improved or cleared up their symptoms in months or even weeks!

Absorption Is Final Key to H2 Water Therapy Success!

Homeostasis is the first key to optimum health. Water & H2 are the keys to homeostasis. Now, let us complete our circle of success by learning how vital absorption is.

We can eat and drink the healthiest food and liquids on earth. But if their nutritional and hydration properties are not fully, completely absorbed by our body, we can still get sick, experience a serious health problem or even have a disease develop inside us. So, how can we best define absorption in terms of "fully and complete?"

Simply put, complete absorption is when our body can absorb via our intestines 100% or nearly 100% of healthy food and liquids. Our digestive system is a marvel of engineering. Its "engineers" should have won the Nobel Prize! Here is how it works with water & H2.

The average American consumes about 2 liters (1/2 Gallon) of water daily through drinking water or via food or other beverages. Also, the volume of gastrointestinal secretions (including salivary, gastric, pancreatic, biliary and intestinal) amounts to around 8 liters (2.1 Gallons), which means that 10 liters (over 2-1/2 Gallons) of water-based fluids enter the intestines every day! [1]

Liquids (without chewing) take the same route as food. We swallow liquids, they pass through our esophagus into our stomach where they wait for our upper intestines to open. Open where? Open via our pyloric valve. The pyloric sphincter (valve) is a thin, circular muscle surrounding the pyloric opening in the first segment (duodenum) of

---

[1] http://www.siumed.edu/mrc/research/nutrient/gi42sg.html

our upper GI tract. Our pyloric valve appears to be pH sensitive and react in a variety of ways under a variety of stomach conditions.

Remember that at least 10 liters (2-1/2 Gallons) of water-based fluids pass through daily! That equals 3,650 liters (912 Gallons) every year! Is our upper GI tract built to process this huge flow? Yes! Our upper intestine is about 20 feet (6 meters) and has an inner surface area of nearly 250 square meters (size of a tennis court)! This large surface is for quick and efficient absorption of water and other fluids. Little wonder our upper intestines absorb about 90% of our water!

However, this next part can be hard to grasp. So, please read it very, very carefully. You may even have to read it twice (LOL). Like all cell membranes, our intestinal cells have a lipid bilayer that is about 5-10 nanometers thick. It is the barrier that marks our cell boundaries. The cell membranes of nearly all living organisms and many viruses are made of a lipid bilayer, as are the membranes surrounding the cell nucleus and other sub-cellular structures. These bilayers are impermeable to most water-soluble (hydrophilic) molecules. Bilayers are particularly impermeable to ions and ionic bonds, which allow cells to regulate salt concentrations and pH by transporting ions across their membranes using proteins called ion pumps.

Most polar molecules (electronegativity between 2 atoms is about 0.5-2.0) have low solubility in the core of a lipid bilayer … and … have low permeability (absorption) characteristics across the bilayer. In this field, biologist and chemists have struggled to understand the complex inner-workings of absorption. So, there are many scientific opinions. The good news is we do not have to figure it out. Why?

Because H2 is the smallest molecule in our known universe and the "purest" covalent bonding non-polar molecule (electronegativity between 2 hydrogen atoms is near 0.0). H2 can safely and easily pass through the lipid bilayer along with healthy water and minerals. This is another "Ah-Ha!" moment for most of us. Why? Because we now have a water that can be fully absorbed at the cellular, sub-cellular, nano and/or epigenetic levels! This is truly NexGen therapy!

Plus, there's research to back this up. One published article shows H2 gas increases gastric emptying (= faster absorption) via increased ghrelin secretion. [1] A clinical study on effects of bicarbonate-alkaline mineral water on gastric functions was more good news. Alkaline mineral water increased gastric emptying (= faster absorption) without changes to healthy mucus linings while simultaneously restoring the stomach's pH back to healthier levels [2] There are more studies.

But do you understand their significance to our NexGen therapy? When we combine the ability of H2 medical gas to safely achieve much faster (and more complete) absorption with the ability of alkaline water to also speed up absorption … we have an unbeatable "team" that can deliver to our bodies all the therapeutic and disease-fighting benefits of "H2 Water 4 Life" therapy!

Are You Excited About This Medical-Science Discovery?

Every month, more global doctors, scientists, researchers and other health professionals embrace H2 water therapy as a great discovery and integrate it into their medical practice and/or personal home health-care program. As we speak with them, hear their lectures or watch their interviews, many speak with passion, enthusiasm, and even excitement about H2 water therapy. This is unusual as most are taught in med school to remain emotionally-neutral. Please notice statements from a few of these experts that may help you understand why we are excited and want others to respond in a similar way.

"All my scientific life has been devoted to heart physiology [heart disease], … I learned about H2 as a potential radical scavenger that could more easily permeate the injured organs; although skeptical, our lab began investigations and were amazed at the protective effects. We did the experiments again and again to confirm the results, as they were difficult to believe. The benefits of hydrogen are more believable now that we know that hydrogen is not simply an

---

[1] https://www.ncbi.nlm.nih.gov/pubmed/16772353 (2006)
[2] https://www.ncbi.nlm.nih.gov/pubmed/12457626 (2002)

antioxidant, ... the clinical applications of hydrogen as a medical gas strongly warrant our further attention." - Dr. Jan Slezak, MD, PhD, D.Sc, Practicing 55 years. Over 57 awards. **Czech Republic**

"Since the discovery of the antioxidant effect of H2 in 2007, we identified the beneficial effects of H2 on mitochondrial respiratory capacity ... which will be [a] very promising molecule in preventing and treating age-related disease and metabolic syndromes." - Dr. Jiangang Long, PhD, (59 Scientific Studies, 2018) Xi'an, **China**

"I witnessed with my own eyes in my own lab the remarkable benefits of hydrogen ... This prompted me to change my research career and surge into hydrogen research. ... my mission [is] to use my expertise in molecular biology to elucidate underlying molecular mechanisms of hydrogen's marked effects and help other people realize the medical benefits of hydrogen gas." – Dr. Kinjo Ohno, MD., PhD., Center for Neurological Diseases & Cancer 2004-Present, **Japan**

"In our published study in PLoS One, Hydrogen Water was remarkable in reversing the various changes induced by controlled cortical impact, an experimental model of traumatic brain injury." – Dr. William A. Banks, 488 Nonabstract Published Manuscripts 1978-2016. Department of Internal Medicine, University of Washington **USA**

"I have been involved with pharmacology for over 30 years. Although hydrogen's effect in Parkinson's disease has now been confirmed in a human clinical trial, more research is necessary ... Because of hydrogen's high safety profile, ease of administration, and its promising medical effects, I feel obligated as a pharmacologist to continue my investigations of H2 as a novel medical gas." – Dr. Mami Noda, PhD, Kyoto Univ. Medical School, 98 Publications 1980-2016, **Japan** [1]

---

[1] http://www.molecularhydrogeninstitute.com/advisory-panel 2018

"Over 200 biomolecules are altered by hydrogen [gas] administration including over 1,000 gene expressions." – MHI, 2018 **(Global)**

Perhaps you now understand why we are convinced that H2 water therapy is the *"greatest discovery in medical-science & health-care since 1953!"* In review, let us summarize its primary benefits:

- Restores homeostasis to our body systems & organs
- Regulates & removes at sub-cellular levels
- Demonstrates highest safety profile
- Prevents or treats hundreds of diseases
- Presents universal approach to personal, home health-care
- Shows no reported noxious side-effects
- Provides a proactive therapy for disease prevention
- Offers fastest & deepest absorption rates
- Supported by a growing global medical & science community

H2 ➡ Homeostasis ➡ Absorption ➡ Optimum Health

H2 infused water has unlimited potential to achieve the above benefits. Clearly, it <u>is</u> the Simplest Solution for Optimum Health!

"You are healthy until you are not healthy." – Ancient Chinese Proverb,
Unknown Source (as best translated into English)

Chapter Sixteen

A Hydrogen Water Therapy System

Before we explain how a home H2 Water Therapy System works, there are some readers who need a little more to reason on. Which readers? In nearly every audience, there are some unusual "older ones" who have lived a wonderful life. Often, they are in their 70s, 80s or even 90s. They are unusual because, presently, their overall health is good. In fact, they may boast that "I haven't been sick for years." … or … "I don't have aches or pains and sleep like a baby." … or … "I may be a little slower, but I am still very mobile and feel great for my age!" For you unusual "older ones" we sincerely have deep respect for you. You have found a way to balance your overall life, including diet and hydration, to achieve a relative homeostasis. However, please read that Proverb again.

"You Are Healthy Until You Are Not Healthy"

What does this Proverb mean? Simply put, we can be healthy one day (for many years or even decades) and that can suddenly change. Another proverb written before 1,000 B.C.E. says about people who are strong or swift: *"time and unexpected events overtake them all."* [1] A car accident, … a slip, trip or fall, … a heavy object falls on us, … we are a victim of crime … a natural disaster, etc. The list is endless. We can suddenly, unexpectedly, be dealing with an older age injury or disease. So, wisdom would have us look ahead and view having a hydrogen water therapy system now like a health insurance policy for our future. Drinking H2 water now would have our older

---

[1] Holy Bible, Hebrew Scriptures ("Old Testament") Ecclesiastes 9:11

bodies in a much stronger condition to endure a sudden injury or disease and potentially recover from it much faster and more completely.

How Does A Home H2 Water Therapy System Work?

There are two "systems" needed, both complimentary to each other, that when properly matched, make a complete high-quality, NexGen home H2 water therapy system. Sadly, we have seen many low-quality or mismatched "systems" that do not perform as advertised.

First, we begin with a pre-ionizer purification system. The expensive approach is to install a whole house filtration system which can cost $5,000 to $10,000. The economical approach is to install a small Point of Delivery (P.O.D.) pre-filter near the water ionizer.

If we choose the pre-filter option, most homes (or other locations) need at least a 2-stage pre-filter with the highest quality parts, best design and most effective medias used to remove "hard-to-remove" contaminants such as arsenic, fluoride, uranium and hexavalent chromium-6. In many homes, a 3 or 4-stage pre-filter will be needed along with a filter cartridge that can either "soften" source water that is "hard" or add minerals to overly soft source water.

Why is making sure we install a quality pre-filter so important? In the U.S., source water for most Americans is so toxic that ionizer filters alone simply cannot remove most of the toxins. If it was built to do so, the ionizer housing (with more filters inside) would be 2 to 3 times larger, would not fit under a sink and be too large for most countertops causing people to decline buying a water ionizer.

How toxic is the source water for most Americans? In most areas, it is contaminated and saturated with poisons, hazardous waste, prescription drugs and Calcium Oxide (CaO) which is quicklime. CaO is a white, caustic (can burn or corrode organic tissue), alkaline, crystalline solid produced by roasting calcium carbonate (very unhealthy) that produces a widely used, inexpensive compound. When mixed with water, CaO causes severe irritation to lungs, skin or eyes. Inhalation may cause labored breathing, pain, nausea and vomiting. Both the Romans & English used clouds of CaO as weapons. Based on research, 50% of manufactured CaO is used in water treatment.

Many systems claim to remove some, most or even 100% of a wide array of contaminants. However, they provide no third-party verification. Thus, it is imperative we verify that a brand of purification medias and/or systems can remove all the contaminants it claims.

Second, we complete our H2 water therapy system with a water ionizer that clearly has a NexGen, innovative design which should be a certified medical device with its own advanced filtration cartridge(s) that complete the purification process.

Source water enters the pre-filter purification stage so that hard-to-remove contaminants are trapped in the pre-filter medias. Next, if necessary, source water is either "softened" or minerals are added in very small amounts. Now our source water is ready to enter a water ionizer. Before it passes over titanium plates dipped or coated in platinum, our source water needs more filtration. A high-quality

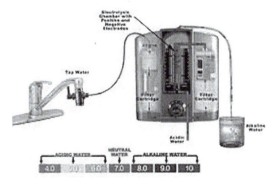

Ionizer example to left is an above counter model. Most companies offer an under counter model that connects directly to cold water valve and hides ionizer unit.

ionizer will have a filter(s) with advanced filtration design, medias and, in some cases, earthen materials to add minerals just before ionization.

What is water ionization? This is where the miracle of molecular hydrogen (H2) is created. Electrolysis is applied to the water passing

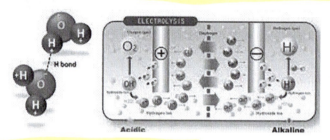

over our titanium/platinum plates. This "ionizes" the water, performing an incredible transformation and splitting of water into two streams. One stream is alkaline, the primary "drinking water" for H2 water therapy. The other stream is acidic and can be used for many other applications that we will not cover in this book.

A Closer Look at H2 Alkaline Water

As previously mentioned, proper pH is an important factor in good health. The pH scale is logarithmic, meaning the difference in 1 pH unit is a difference of 10 times! If any substance changes from pH 7.0 to pH 8.0 it becomes ten times more alkaline. Conversely, if it changes from neutral pH 7.0 down to pH 6.0 it is ten times more acidic. For example, a soda pop at 2.5 pH is almost 50,000 times more acidic than 7.0 pH neutral water. However, a more emphatic example would be going from drinking healthy 9.5 pH alkaline water to drinking that same soda pop at 2.5 pH acidity. That one can or bottle of soda pop would be 10,000,000 times more acidic! Of course, our

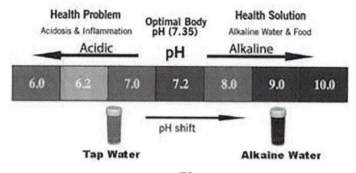

well-designed stomach digestive system can adjust to this anomaly on occasion. So, we are not suggesting that one can of soda pop is going to kill you. But our illustration should be obvious. A regular, continued consumption of highly acidic beverages could and probably would negate most of the beneficial alkaline properties of H2 water. Also, please understand that our blood pH can be affected at any time by food, water, beverages, events, stress, pollution, trauma, exercise and many other things.

The next benefit of drinking freshly-ionized H2 alkaline water is it contains millions of antioxidants! We need to flood our bodies with an abundance of antioxidants. Why? Most of us understand that excessive oxidation in our bodies is harmful. Oxidative stress, when left to run wild inside our bodies for weeks, months or even years will often lead to serious health problems and diseases. It is vital to help our bodies' need to balance oxidation (such as its need for oxygen, nitric oxide, etc.) with anti-oxidation. Again, as with alkaline, this one area of balance is part of an overall attempt to achieve homeostasis.

H2 is unique among all antioxidants in that it is a weak antioxidant that is selective and therefore does not interfere or neutralize important reactive oxygen species (ROS). The most effective, efficient and expedient way to deliver this superior antioxidant is by daily drinking many glasses of freshly-ionized H2 alkaline water that contains millions of antioxidants in every glass!

Antioxidants can be measured using an ORP meter. ORP stands for oxidation reduction potential. On an ORP chart, the +ORP (plus) numbers are oxidative and the -ORP (negative) numbers are anti-oxidative. Notice the chart:

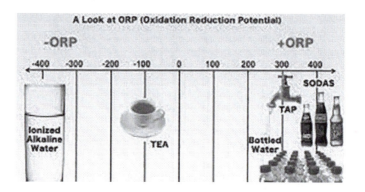

A Look at ORP (Oxidation Reduction Potential)

Excessive oxidation is how our bodies age resulting in wrinkles, degeneration of organs, bones, muscles, tendons and cellular membranes. An anti-oxidant reducing agent is simply something that inhibits or slows the process of oxidation.

The +ORP of most tap water in the USA is between +200 to +300mV and so is an oxidizing agent. Most bottled waters are both acidic and have higher +ORP's, making them increase our internal oxidation. Sodas, sports & energy drinks can be even worse! Some of these have acidic pH as low as 2.5 pH (car battery acid is 1.0 pH) and are extremely oxidizing with +ORP readings as high as +550mV!

The *most important benefit of drinking H2 Water is,* of course, the molecular hydrogen gas. Studies using dissolved hydrogen in water range from 0.5 mg/L to 1.6+ mg/L, with most using 1.6 mg/L (1.6 ppm). A high-quality water ionizer should produce a therapeutic dose of 0.5 mg/L (0.5 ppm) to 1.6 mg/L (1.6 ppm) depending on its power setting or capacity in relation to its progressive alkaline levels.

In some early human studies where 1-3 mg/L of H2 were administered, these doses showed significant health benefits. So, for most of us it is a matter of drinking a larger quantity of H2 water versus convenience or desire to drink a larger quantity. For some, this may be a matter of choice or circumstance due to personal limitations or travel considerations. But let's do the math:

- 1 liter = 33.8 ounces (slightly over a quarter-gallon)

- We would have to drink 3 liters (over 3/4-gallon) to reach 3 mg (3.0 ppm) for faster and/or significant health benefits

Some choose to drink 3 liters of H2 water (over 3/4-gallon). Others choose or have no choice but to use portable devices/products such as hydrogen generators or tablets that can add about 1.0 ppm, usually based on a 500 ml amount of water. But remember that portable devices or tablets *do not filter the water.* They can only add a therapeutic dose of H2 medical gas, usually in about 5 minutes. Portable devices and products can never replace a complete hydrogen water therapy system that has filters to remove hundreds of contaminants.

Is more H2 better? Early studies appear to say yes! And it also appears you cannot get too much H2. Why? Because it does not build up in our bodies. We simply exhale any excess. So, in many cases, the more hydrogen the better! Of course, health benefits will vary widely from person to person and more research needs to be done.

More Good Things to Know About H2 Water

- ❖ Does H2 escape from the water? Yes. But no need to worry. Under standard ambient temperature & pressure (SATP) along with surface area, agitation, etc., when H2 in water is held in a 500 ml container (or a large, open glass) and exposed to air, it has a half-life of about 2 hours. So, no need to hurry.

- ❖ Drinking a therapeutic dose of H2 Water via at least one glass (8 ounces) but preferably 500 ml (16.9 ounces) results in a peak rise in plasma and breath concentration in as little as 5 to 15 minutes. Depending on dosage, return to baseline will be in 45 to 90 minutes.

- ❖ Early research shows that H2 has a residual effect that continues improving health or disease symptoms up to 4 weeks.

- ❖ Drinking 1 to 2 glasses (8 to 16 ounces) after sleeping 6 to 8 hours replenishes our body's reserves and primes our digestive tract for breakfast.

- ❖ Drinking 1 or 2 glasses before a main meal curbs our tendency to overeat. When water is consumed before a meal we tend to chew more completely, rather than washing food down.

- ❖ H2 Water is a perfect delivery fluid (and system) when taking nutritional supplements. It can ensure maximum absorption!

Do All of Us Need a Hydrogen Water Therapy System?

We will let a global institute of doctors and scientists help us answer that question by sharing some human studies they conducted. [1]

"Clinical studies suggest that ingestion of hydrogen-rich water was beneficial for"

- Metabolic Syndrome [71]
- Diabetes [72]
- Hyperlipidemia [73, 74]
- Parkinson's Disease [75]
- Rheumatoid Arthritis [24, 76]
- Mitochondrial Dysfunction [77]
- Exercise Performance [78]
- Athletic Recovery Time [79]
- Wound Healing [80-82]
- Oxidative stress reduction from Chronic Hepatitis B [83]
- Blood Flow Improvements [84]
- Periodontitis Improvements [85]
- Dialysis [86, 87]
- Patients receiving Radiotherapy [Radiation] for Tumors [88]

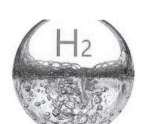

"Give me good digestion, Lord, and also something to digest; but where and how [it] comes I leave to Thee, who knoweth best." – Mary Webb novelist & Poet

Chapter Seventeen

When to Drink H2 Water & Eat Meals

Below are beginner guidelines to increase our H2 water therapy benefits, improve digestion and better manage or lose weight. Our goal is to simplify drinking and eating so we can enjoy both with ease.

MORNING: When we wake up, drink 500 ml (2 x 8 oz glasses = 16 oz.) of freshly-ionized H2 alkaline water on an empty stomach. Each time we drink 1 or 2 glasses of H2 alkaline water, wait 20 minutes. Why? Because we must allow our pH-sensitive pyloric valve to open wide and let this very safe medical-grade water to quickly flow through our valve into our upper GI tract (upper intestines). TIP: 20 minutes after drinking our 1st 16 oz. (2 glasses) on empty stomach, we drink a 2nd 16 oz. (2 glasses) of fresh H2 water. This gives us a daily 1-quarter gallon "foundation" of H2 gas & micro-minerals that is alive in alkaline water with millions of antioxidants!

Why is the 20-Minute Wait Guideline So Important?

We always want to separate putting too much water in our stomach from putting food in our stomach at the same time. Our stomach and pyloric valve have well-designed "sensor" mechanisms with very intelligent feedback loops. When our stomach senses any food, it immediately interprets that food as a meal and produces acids to digest our "meal" … even if it is only a snack.

VERY IMPORTANT NOTE: Drinking high-alkaline water with a meal or too soon after a meal can have a negative impact on our stomach's ability to efficiently digest food. Remember … we need our stomach to be acidic for healthy digestion! So, if we must drink water with our meal, we drink just a little bit of pH neutral purified "H2O" water from our ionizer that removes hundreds of contaminants.

How Long Do We Wait After a Snack or Meal?

It is vital to allow our stomach enough time to digest food using its well-designed digestive system. Our stomach must remain acidic for healthy digestion. Thus, *we do not drink lots of water with any meal.* This will hinder digestion. If we must drink to swallow a pill or a portion of our food, drink just a little (sip). Alcohols like wine and beer are acidic. So, alcohols are OK to slowly drink (sip) before, with or after a meal in moderation. Many cultures enjoy wine, beer or other alcohols with a main meal and are often very healthy!

- After a **light snack or meal**: Wait 1 hour for your stomach to digest food. After this, drink 1 or 2 glasses of H2 water
- After an **average-size meal**: Wait 2 hours for your stomach to digest food. After this, drink 1 or 2 glasses of H2 water
- After a **heavy meal** (especially with hard-to-digest proteins like red meat): Wait 3 hours. Then resume H2 hydration.

Do you see how simple drinking and eating can be? We call this our easy **20-Minute / 1-2-3 Method**. First, we wait 20 minutes each time we drink H2 alkaline water before drinking or eating anything else. Second, depending on the size of our meal, we wait 1, 2 or 3 hours before drinking H2 alkaline water again.

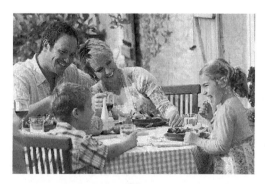

"The more research that accumulates about [H2], the more it appears to have the … properties of the Fountain of Youth." – Molecular Hydrogen Institute, 2018

Chapter Eighteen

Ionized H2 Water – What to Expect

The first thing that ionized H2 water does when we begin drinking it is flush out our digestive tract, which is the best place to start detoxification. This cleansing alone will significantly improve our potential for better health. Our body cannot take in nutrients if our digestive tract is not clean. Enzymes continue their chemical attack on the food to break it down throughout our digestive process until it is small enough to pass through the lining of our small intestine and into our blood. Once there, nutrients are carried to our liver and other body parts to be processed, stored and distributed. Little to none of this happens if our digestive tract is not clean of waste and debris.

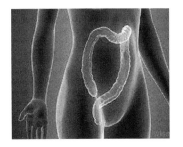

DETOXIFYING. Our intestines can become museums of partially digested, putrefied foods, drugs and other toxins that never found their way out of our body. If our small (upper) intestines are not clean and their wall lining is not exposed, nutrients cannot get into our blood stream for our body to use. Ionized H2 water is a terrific cleanser of our digestive tract because tiny nano-size bubbles (dissolved molecular hydrogen gas) can be infused into the water by an ionizer. Plus, H2 gently cleans our GI tract while it also hydrates our tract's lining, so nutrients can pass into our blood with greater ease.

When this occurs, assimilation of nutrients into our body returns and early stages of cellular rejuvenation can begin. When first drinking ionized H2 water, people comment how often they go to the bathroom. This is GOOD because H2 water is fully cleansing our digestive tract, organs, joints, tissues, nerves, skin and bones! It will subside after our body is used to drinking H2 water every day.

ALKALIZING. Drinking H2 alkaline water reduces our body's overall acid level as it balances our body's overall pH, which is best measured through our urine or saliva. However, raising our overall body pH will most likely take some time. Acid waste did not accumulate throughout our body overnight and it will not be flushed out overnight. Many years of accumulated acid waste in our joints, around our organs, in our brain and throughout our body takes months and even years to completely expunge. Of course, … how quickly we cleanse our body of acid waste also depends on our diet.

OXYGENATING. All bodily functions depend on oxygen for cellular respiration. Our cells mainly need oxygen for two functions: 1) to produce ATP; 2) to eliminate toxins and waste through oxidation. Our lungs consume about 5-6 milligrams per minute and we breathe about 17,000-30,000 times per day. Through our lungs, oxygen enters a capillary network and is bonded to hemoglobin (a protein molecule in red blood cells). Our red blood cells transport oxygen. Each one contains about 270 million oxygen-binding hemoglobin molecules. If blood circulation is poor, oxygen delivery is reduced. When viewed under a microscope, conventional water moves our red blood cells slowly. In contrast, H2 water moves our red blood cells rapidly throughout our body. So, drinking ionized H2 water can increase our blood oxygen delivery, energy levels and elimination of toxins.

ANTIOXIDANT. There is a constant battle inside our body between elements that are oxidative and antioxidant. H2 water is rich in antioxidants and bathes our body in the lightest liquid for human

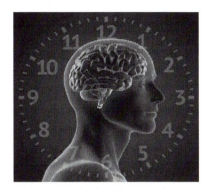

consumption. H2 promotes rejuvenation of each bodily system at a sub-cellular level. Plus, H2 triggers activation or upregulation of antioxidant enzymes (glutathione, superoxide dismutase, catalase, etc.)

Antioxidants are associated with anti-aging. H2 gas has antioxidant properties. We can slow down and/or reverse aging by drinking ionized H2 water. However, we do not become younger in chronological years. If we are 40 years old, we do not become 20 again. Rather, we can possess the body we had when we were in our twenties at a cellular level. The cells that make up our body can be as active, productive, functional and communicative as those we had in our prime. Thus, we have reversed our biological clock, not our chronological clock. Like an older home that needs remodeling, our body can gradually be "remodeled" to feel like its younger self … month-by-month, year-by-year as we daily drink plenty of H2 water.

HYDRATING. After we drink ionized H2 water for a while, we become more sensitive to when we are dehydrated. For example, we become aware that our body needs water after only an hour of not

drinking any water. By keeping our body constantly hydrated, we accomplish many things that are necessary to achieve great health. Staying hydrated with H2 water helps stave off disease better than anything else we can do. When we are hydrated, our blood is never too thin nor too thick due to lack of water or salt. Most of us do not

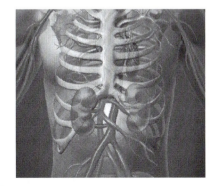

retain salt nor have high blood pressure when we drink plenty of healthy H2 water. Our organs function optimally because they are not starved for water, especially our kidneys.

Like any muscle, regular use of our kidneys will strengthen them. A common misconception is that drinking too much water can overtax our kidneys. If you have weak kidneys from dehydration or living on a nutrient-poor diet, start by drinking freshly-ionized H2 alkaline water with a 7.5 to 8.5 pH. When we provide our body with a full array of nutrients from real foods and drink plenty of H2 alkaline water, our weak kidneys can become powerful, flexing muscles again. This is true of any muscle or organ in our body.

BENEFITS. The benefits of H2 water are overwhelming! Please examine the following chart that includes just some of these:

BENEFITS	H2 Alkaline Water	Bottle Water (Plastic)	Tap Water	Well Water
Antioxidants	YES	NO	NO	NO
Balance Body pH	YES	NO	NO	NO
Powerful Detoxifier	YES	NO	NO	NO
Superior Hydrator	YES	NO	NO	NO
Best Mineral Absorption	YES	NO	NO	NO
Increased Oxygen	YES	NO	NO	NO

In 2015, Dr. Shigeo Ohta, Dept. of Biochemistry & Cell Biology, wrote Molecular Hydrogen as a Novel Antioxidant, Advantages for Medical Applications in which he stated with conviction: *"H2 rapidly diffuses into tissues and cells. ... We propose H2 for prevention and therapeutic applications ... for many diseases."*

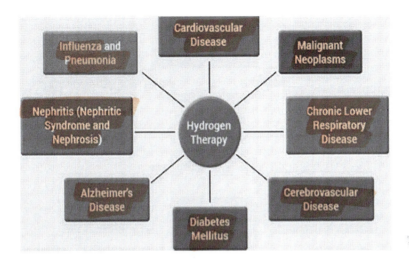

Everyone's body has various degrees of toxicity. Therefore, the effects of H2 water on our body will be different than everyone else. It will depend on our past and current diet, how much water we drink, how much we exercise, how positive we are, how stressful our life is, how much medicine we took in the past or take now, and how toxic we are. Regardless of the above, H2 water can be LIFE-CHANGING or even LIFE-SAVING for all of us who drink it every day!

"Pets are humanizing. They remind us we have an obligation to preserve and nurture and care for all life." – James Cromwell, actor & animal lover.

Chapter Nineteen

What About Our Pets?

Most pet owners hydrate their animals with dead, acidic and/or toxic water containing hundreds of contaminants. So, let us rethink what we give our precious pets to drink. First, we need to learn a little about their unique bodies.

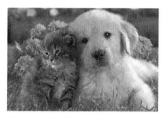

Dogs have a warmer body temperature of 101 to 102.5 degrees Fahrenheit. Cats also have a warmer temperature of 99.5-102.5 and are prone to pyrexia, a fever of at least 103.5 that can be deadly. Keeping pets fully hydrated, especially during heat waves, is vital. Giving our pets H2 water can easily do this and might just save their lives!

Is H2 water safe for smaller pets? Yes. However, we need to match alkaline level and hydrogen potency to animal size.

- o Small pets: alkaline 7.5-8.5 pH / H2 0.5 ppm (+/- 0.1)
- o Medium pets: alkaline 8-9 pH / H2 1.0 ppm (+/- 0.2)
- o Large pets or animals (like horses): 9-10 pH / H2 1.6 ppm

Will H2 water shock my pet's body? It could if we start our pet on too high a level. So, we begin on the mildest level. Then gradually increase their quantity and levels to match their size.

Can H2 water help older pets with severe health problems? Yes. The sooner we put our beloved pet on H2 water therapy, its potential for relieving our pet's suffering can begin. Most pets are mammals just like us. So, the amazing antioxidant properties of H2 that help humans can aid our pet's digestive and immune systems.

There is much more to learn about H2 water therapy for pets that we can cover in a separate book. For now, next to our love and care, H2 water could be the greatest gift we ever give to our precious pets and animals!

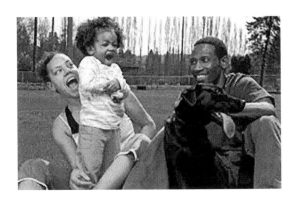

"Football is like life – it requires perseverance, self-denial, hard work, sacrifice, dedication and respect for authority." – Vince Lombardi, NFL Coach

Chapter Twenty

Pro Athletes – This One Is For You!

Steven has been a Pro Football fan since the 1960s. He still remembers watching the first Super Bowl on January 15, 1967 … on his parents black & white console TV from Sears. He memorized key details such as the game was played at L.A. Memorial Coliseum and attendance was 61,946 with over 51,000,000 watching on TVs. He knows the Green Bay Packers beat the Kansas City Chiefs 35-10 with coach Vince Lombardi as the mastermind and quarterback Bart Starr leading their team to victory! [1] So, this chapter is written from a very sincere mind & heart.

Most pro athletes live, work and perform in a fast-pace, highly-competitive and very stressful world. Each week, they push their bodies far beyond what is normal to most of us. For NFL pro football players, this begins the first week of August with pre-season games and continues through the last week in December for 22 weeks in a row, having only one week off as a "bye" week! Let's look closer.

First, most National Football League (NFL) pro players work 6 days a week. Even when they are home with their families, their "rest" and "private" time is limited because performing at their level requires focus, study, learning hundreds of plays and following a strict workout, diet and hydration routine.

Second, pro NFL players earn above average salaries. In 2018, the minimum 1-year contract for a rookie is $480,000. There are only

---

[1] https://www.nfl.com/super-bowl/history/1967

1,656 active players at any given time. So, they live in a world that is highly-competitive among players who know there is always another player waiting to take their position. This is very stressful!

Third, perhaps what causes all pro athletes (in all pro sports) the most worry and anxiety is the real possibility of a career-ending injury. The risk of this happening to a pro NFL player is extremely high because they perform in a very high-contact sport. During a game, pro football plays and players move at incredible speeds. So, a freak injury to a primary joint, their spine or a brain concussion can occur at any moment! Their health & quality of life permanently changed.

Now, let us take just a glimpse into their dedication to excellence by examining the routine of a pro NFL player. But please keep in mind a version of their routine is duplicated in most other high-contact pro sports.

An Average Week in the Life of a Pro NFL Player

After their Sunday game, a pro NFL player will usually have only one day off on Tuesday. The other six days will be filled with exhaustion, dehydration, injury evaluations, weight-lifting, workouts, calorie-count postings, watching film, real on-field practices, media interviews and multiple recoveries. Let us look at one of their busiest days, Wednesday, knowing that a variation of it occurs on other days.

- 6:00 am: Cafeteria opens.
- 7:00 am: Weight-lifting
- 8:00-11:15 am: Meetings, learn plays, watch film, etc.
- 11:45 am – 1:45 pm: On-field practice
- 1:30-2:15 pm: Media sessions (on field or in locker room)
- 2:30-5:00 pm: More meetings
- 5:00-7:00 pm: Dinner
- 7:00 pm: Players may leave. Most bring their tablet computers home to study game film later that night

Many pro NFL players go to bed between 10:00-11:00 pm. That is almost 16 hours of their minds focused on learning complex plays and their bodies enduring the physical challenges of real contact on-field practices. This is repeated for 22 consecutive weeks!

Clearly, pro athletes (especially pro NFL players) are submerged in a world that most of us cannot begin to fathom. Perhaps this glimpse can help most of us to develop a deeper respect for their chosen profession.

Pro Athletes & H2 Water

The greatest worry for all pro athletes is a major injury to their spine, a limb, bone, joint, knee, hip or shoulder. Fortunately, H2 water can potentially rescue our dedicated athletes from such career-ending injuries. There are also 7 other areas of concern for pro athletes:

- Maximum oxygen uptake
- Reliable, consistent energy levels
- Muscle fatigue
- Lactic acid build-up
- Faster post-workout or post-game recoveries
- Inflammation
- Micro-injuries to bones, joints, muscles, connective tissues and nerves, including brain tissues & nerves

We have access to many scientific studies on these 7 areas of concern. One published in 2012 was a human study of elite male soccer players. [1] This real, in-the-field human study concluded, in part, that adequate H2 hydration *"pre-exercise reduced blood lactate levels and improved exercise-induced decline of muscle fatigue."*

It is no longer theory that H2 water therapy can, in most cases, prevent or treat all 7 areas pro athletes constantly worry about. Just imagine, as a pro athlete, knowing you have, perhaps, the ultimate edge in your category of sports. Imagine, waking up every day with a confidence,

---

[1] https://www.ncbi.nlm.nih.gov/pubmed/22520831

knowing your hydration protocol is backed by over 1,000 scientific studies proving H2 Water is protecting, repairing and delivering therapeutic properties to your entire body at a nano level!

Every month, more pro athletes are adding H2 water to their hydration program. Some of the biggest names in pro sports already have an H2 edge. However, without proper education/training by a Certified Molecular Hydrogen Advisor and Nano Hydration Specialist … *most athletes may experience no more than 50% of its benefits.*

There are very specific dosage protocols for pro athletes that should be customized to each individual athlete. Upon request, we can provide more research and/or free classes for any single pro athlete or group of pro athletes, including entire teams of elite athletes.

"When you're young, you don't think very far ahead. You just think in terms of the next day, the next week, the next competition. You don't think about injuries that could threaten your long-term health." – Katarina Witt, Figure Skater, Gold Medalist

Chapter Twenty-One

Add H2 Therapy to High-Contact Pro Sports Injury & Concussion Protocols

The above quote says it all. It's time for pro athletes world-wide, especially those in high-contact pro sports, to embrace a Global Movement towards injury prevention via H2 Water Therapy. The research and scientific evidence are both irrefutable and undeniable. A massive body of studies that span over 40 years indicates that a NexGen therapy with virtually universal applications for all pro sports is available today! So, we propose that H2 therapy be added as a primary adjunct to existing injury and concussion protocols … at all levels of high-contact sports, including public & private school programs.

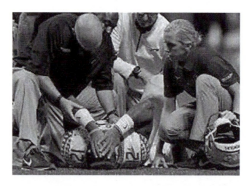

The above image is a painful reminder that injuries and concussions happen every week in the tens of thousands around the globe. These injuries impact our young children, teenagers, college athletes and pro

athletes. But for meaningful change to occur, the focus on profits needs to be put on hold. Leaders on both sides of high-contact sports should be open to examining H2 therapy. Why? Because there is virtually nothing to lose and essentially unlimited benefits to gain. Let us briefly examine those benefits.

Unlimited Benefits to Implement H2 Therapy into All Sports

In Chapter 17, we outlined 7 main concerns for pro athletes. Let us now take one giant step further. Today, we have so many peer-reviewed scientific studies that demonstrate a wide range of therapeutic benefits to the sports world. Let us zero in on brain concussions.

One break-through study on Traumatic Brain Injury (TBI) stated that *"acute TBI can transform into a chronic condition and be a risk factor for diseases such as Alzheimer's and Parkinson's."* It listed many serious TBI conditions that H2 therapy could more quickly reverse. In closing, the 11 highly-respected doctors and/or scientists stated with total confidence that molecular hydrogen water *"could be an easily administered, highly-effective treatment for TBI."* [1]

How many of us have seen former pro athletes develop these horrible brain disorders in their 60s, 50s or even 40s? A prime example is the famous NFL Hall of Fame Quarterback, Brett Favre, who is only 48-years-old. He was diagnosed with Chronic Traumatic Encephalopathy (CTE) by Dr. Bennet Omalu. In 2010, Favre's career came to an end during a game when his head hit the frozen turf. There are 4 stages to this degenerative disease. According to Dr. Omalu, Favre shows symptoms of Stage 1 and/or Stage 2 which include short-term memory lapses and difficulty in speech. Favre admits that his

---

[1] Doji, K., et al., Molecular Hydrogen in Drinking Water Protects against Neurodegenerative Changes Induced by Traumatic Brain Injury. *PLoS*, 2014
http://www.molecularhydrogeninstitute.com/brain
https://www.ncbi.nlm.nih.gov/pubmed/25251220

brain injuries are *"a part of my future that I really can't control and that is very scary."* [1]

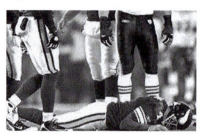

Prevention and treatment of degenerative diseases from brain concussion via H2 water therapy is available today. But the bigger picture includes all the benefits of H2 water applied toward keeping athletes at a superior level of health pre-injury, during injury treatment or surgery, and post-injury rehab/recovery. Reduction of expenses coupled with savings in time, lost talent, insurance costs along with increasing maximum performance could potentially save all sports leagues and organizations a combined amount into the billions of dollars!

- Reduction of overall expenses
- Less minor injuries and less major injuries
- Savings in time, lost talent, insurance costs and other areas
- Increasing maximum performance of athletes
- Improved public and player/league relations & image
- Combined leagues/organizations savings – billions of dollars!
- Superior level of health for athletes' pre-injury, during injury treatment or surgery, and post-injury rehab & recovery

We invite leaders from every level of sports leagues and/or organizations to consider the risk to reward. There is virtually little to no risk to begin adding, even on a trial basis, H2 therapy to existing injuries and concussion protocols. The reward is essentially unlimited potential preventive and treatment benefits for all athletes.

---

[1] www.washingtonpost.com/news/early-lead/wp/2018/04/12/brett-favre-says-he-suffered-probably-thousands-of-concussions/
https://en.wikipedia.org/wiki/Chronic_traumatic_encephalopathy

The purpose of this chapter is to lay out an invitation from a global community of highly-respected doctors, scientists and medical researchers to transform the world of high-contact sports into a much safer workplace for all athletes to perform. Therefore, we stand ready to educate and help integrate H2 water therapy into any level or size of sports leagues and/or organizations for the benefit of all parties.

To review more scientific studies that apply to the world of all pro sports, please visit the worldwide non-profit organization below that is leading this NexGen global movement into H2 water therapy. After your review, please contact H2 WATER 4 LIFE via the email address below to begin a dialogue with us.

www.molecularhydrogeninstitute.com/studies

info@h2water4life.com

"He that Hath a truth and keeps it, keeps what not to him belongs. But performs a selfish action, And a fellow mortal wrongs." – Andrew Jackson David

Chapter Twenty-Two

What People are Saying About a Hydrogen Water Therapy System - Testimonials

Because a Hydrogen Water Therapy System can rejuvenate our body, practitioners and their patients who use H2 water therapy have reported numerous benefits: Some reports include the ability to:

* Reduce chronic pain
* Release excess body fat and stored toxins
* Normalize blood pressure
* Support healthy colon function
* Normalize blood sugar and insulin
* Resolve urinary tract infections
* Relieve asthma and chronic respiratory infections
* Stop abnormal gastro-intestinal putrefaction
* Improve wound healing
* Reduce proliferation of candida

Many people are achieving wondrous results using a hydrogen water therapy system. There are devices in the market place claiming to be great systems. But a high-quality system is different because it is designed with its specific purpose already determined. Plus, it is based on solid medical research. A high-quality system utilizes the most up-to-date, cutting edge technology to ensure a safe, consistent and therapeutic dose of H2 (Molecular Hydrogen) gas is safely infused into our water each time, when proper maintenance and cleaning are performed at recommended intervals.

A Few User Testimonials

Dementia, Depression, Positive Attitude & More Energy

"In 2016, I found out about ionized, alkaline H2 water through a friend. He invited my wife, Rondi, & I to a water learning party in his home. The teacher drove over 800 miles to teach our little group. At that time, I was 78 and Rondi was 74. She was showing signs of Dementia, had depression, barely communicating and was tired all the time. We were amazed at what we learned and I immediately ordered 2 ionizer systems. He installed our system 3 days later. We progressed to level 3 alkaline with more hydrogen by week 9. She drank a minimum of 6 glasses a day; most days at least 8 glasses. Four months later, my wife was a new person. I called the H2 teacher to joyfully report that her dementia was greatly improved (memories returning), she was no longer depressed, her positive attitude returned, she was like a 'chatter-box' compared to before, we were having conversations again and she had more energy. About a year ago, her doctor did diagnose her with dementia. However, we are hopeful that if we increase her daily intake of hydrogen with H2 tablets, she will experience even faster results."
– *Larry E., Spokane Washington*

Family Shielded From Sickness & Diseases

"Last year, I heard about ionized H2 water from a friend. So, our family started drinking H2 water daily. We were already healthy. But prevention/protection are better than treatment. Last winter, every family in our circle of friends with young children went down with multiple bouts of sickness. Many became sick three or four times! My child was shielded from both sickness and diseases while drinking H2 water every day, even though he was in the same rooms as children who were sick. We are grateful to have our health and not miss work or the things we love. Perhaps our story will inspire more families to enjoy the same health benefits." – **Rev. Andria S., MD Univ. of Chicago, B.A. Univ. of Oregon, Rockford Illinois**

Severe Weight Loss, Chronic Fatigue, Arthritis, Decision-Function & Dogs Love It!

"In 2014, my dear husband, Gaston, suffering from extreme fatigue, stress, high-anxiety and insomnia. He took prescribed medication to sleep. Results? Horror! Severe weight Loss: 35 pounds in 6 weeks, Chronic Fatigue, complete muscular loss, severe Arthritis, & decision-function loss. I did research and found water ionizer technology as a safe, alternative therapy. We bought our first of 3 ionizers. Immediately, we saw a difference: ionized water was lighter & tasteless. Eventually, Gaston was able to drink from a better ionizer brand that produced about 1.0 ppm of H2 at its highest alkaline level. His health problems rapidly improved and today are virtually gone! H2 water is a daily part of our lives and even our beloved dogs love it! I thank God for this priceless gift. What a blessing!" – **Guylaine D., Québec Canada**

Type 2 Diabetes

"In 2016, I was diagnosed with Type 2 Diabetes and my doctor immediately put me on meds to control it. A friend (Emma) told me about how her H2 water system helped her overcome many serious health problems. So, I attended a free H2 class. In October 2016 the class instructor installed my 4 filter water purifying & ionizing system. He encouraged me to drink a minimum of 64 oz (1/2 gallon) daily, but try to drink 1 full gallon for faster results. So, most days I drank a gallon of H2 water. 3 weeks and 5 days later, I went to my doctor to review my lab tests. My doctor was surprised that my Hemoglobin A1C test was down to 86 and my Fasting Plasma Glucose test was below 100! So, my doctor took me off my meds and advised me to monitor my levels at home to make sure they stay below 100. I immediately called the class instructor with my exciting news. As of April 2018 I've been med-free for almost 1-1/2 years! Thank you hydrogen water therapy!" – *Portia S., Rio Vista California*

Rotator Cuff Disorder, More Energy & Look Younger

"In July 2016 I learned about ionized alkaline H2 water. I was 75-years-old, having severe pain in my rotator cuff and 'pooped out' every day by 1:00 pm. My wife and I attended a free H2 water wellness party where we saw a beautiful water dispenser attached above the kitchen sink and asked about it. The host served us some level 1 H2 water and we tasted the difference immediately. It was light and did not give us that bloated feeling in our stomachs. The party was so much fun, we won prizes and were impressed at how much we learned in just a couple hours. It was an easy decision to buy our own filtration and ionizer system. I was facing surgery on my rotator cuff. But I chose to start with physical therapy (PT) that my surgeon said would take 6 to 8 months. I began drinking about 12 to 16 glasses of fresh H2 water daily. Within one month, I noticed the pain was nearly gone. After 2 months of drinking H2 water, I was on level 3 (about 1.0 ppm of H2) and my pain was completely gone! I discontinued my PT. So, combining H2 water therapy with physical therapy cut that time by two-thirds (2/3). I am now 77-years-old, have tons of energy and people think I'm in my 60s." – *Ted L., Knoxville Tennessee*

Over 20 Years of Migraines, High Blood Pressure & Pain Issues
"In 2017, I heard about the health benefits of hydrogen alkaline water. For over 20 years, I suffered with migraines, and later developed high blood pressure and pain issues. So, I bought my first ionizer system. In about 2 months, when I reached level 3 alkaline with more H2 in the water, my migraines were gone! As I kept drinking at least 8 to 10 glasses a day, I was better able to manage my blood pressure and pain problems. The only time I am sad is when I am away from my ionizer system for a long time and have to drink bottled water, like now, I am working in another country." – *Julita W., Las Vegas Nevada & Pyeongtaek South Korea*

Quest for Water, Energized, Better Skin & No More Tooth Infections!
"My mission is health through Biblical Wellness. The holy books taught me about the importance of healthy food and water, mentioning water 722 times! I tried all types of water systems and none were meeting my standards for optimum health. My quest for the healthiest water finally brought me to a free H2 water wellness video-slideshow class in Florida. After listening to our instructor articulate his years of research on water, including the discovery of hydrogen as a medical gas with limitless therapeutic potential, I knew my journey was over. I purchased a very advanced combo 4-filter ionizer system that day. I finally found the 'Fountain' of Youth.' Two days later, our class instructor installed my countertop system. In the biblical sense, 'Water is our Well for Wellness.' Natural water has two critical elements for life, hydrogen and oxygen, both vital for maximizing energy. I am amazed how energized I feel, how my skin feels and looks. I had some teeth issues, getting infections routinely. Since rinsing every morning with fresh, ionized water, I have not had one infection in over a year. I am now drinking the best water on earth! As a health-care professional, I feel confident referring my clients to our instructor and H2 Water 4 Life!" - *Reverend Kathryn M., D.D., M.S., Licensed Nurse & Educator, Seminole Florida*

Open Heart Surgery, Severe Dehydration & Memories at 94-Years-Old
"I've been drinking ionized alkaline water for many years. In 2015, I helped my 92-year-old father get an ionizer. He recently had open heart surgery and was dealing with high blood pressure, pneumonia, weak lungs, low energy and dehydration. After drinking about 8 glasses a day and working up to alka level 3 (about 9.5pH), my Dad's blood pressure, breathing, hydration and skin elasticity significantly improved. He also resumed his daily walks. To my sadness, Dad gradually slowed down his alkaline water intake until he suddenly complained to my siblings (who are his loving care-givers) that

he was dizzy and felt like he was going to faint. They rushed Dad to E.R. He was diagnosed with severe dehydration. I found out Dad was only drinking 3 cups (not glasses) of alkaline water daily. I explained to Dad and my family that DAD HAS THE BEST WATER IN THE WORLD & MUST DRINK AT LEAST 8 GLASSES A DAY TO AVOID DEHYDRATION. A key to getting Dad to drink more was offering him flavored electrolytes. 3 months later my Dad was back to his 2016 better health. During a private visit, I was amazed to hear my 94-year-old Dad's memories come back, telling me stories about his childhood, his teenage years, his time in the Navy, all with specific details! My Dad also wanted to know the details of his credit card and bank account balances to make decisions again like he did when he was 92-years-old." – *Christina C. P. C., Ceres California*

Squamous Skin Cell Carcinoma (Cancer) & No Negative Side-Effects

"I was 70-years-old in November 2014 when I was first diagnosed with squamous cell tumors. My doctor immediately ordered a parotidectomy to remove the cancer tumors and put me on radiation treatments. In April 2015 a biopsy of my eyelid confirmed the 1st surgery failed and my skin cancer was rapidly spreading. So, a 2nd surgery was needed to remove my left eye. In January 2017 a 3rd surgery was performed to remove cancerous cells that came back to my neck. Sadly, all three surgeries, radiation and meds failed. By September 2017 I had a "ping-pong ball" size tumor pushing out my neck with purple discoloration and radiation burns. A loving neighbor (Lupe) told us about H2 hydrogen water that I should immediately begin. My wife, Eleanor, & I contacted a certified molecular hydrogen advisor. He invited us to his home for a simplified version of his H2 water therapy class that same day! On the next day, he personally installed our 4-filter water purification & ionizer system! Because I had an aggressive cancer, after 2 days, I advanced to alka level 2, and 2 days later to alka level 3 with no discomfort, no negative side-effects. When home, I was drinking 1 to 1-1/2 gallons daily to get maximum H2 into my cells. Within 3 weeks, my skin color was lighter. After 3 months of H2 alkaline water, the ping-pong ball tumor disappeared and the cancer looked like it was gone. About 1 month later, a PET scan confirmed that this cancer appeared to be gone from my neck." – *Robert R., Rio Vista California*

Acid Reflux, Stamina & Severe Acne

I suffered for decades with acid reflux, taking 2 pills a day. In 2017, I bought my first ionizer, stopped drinking sodas, and drank a gallon every day of highly-filtered alkaline H2 water only. In about one week, my painful digestive problem cleared up – no more acid reflux & no more pills! Before

H2 water, I was wiped out by afternoon due to my fast-pace field job. Today, at 54-years-old, I have more stamina drinking hydrogen water all day. My adult son suffered for years with severe acne. His face was covered in red swelling and large painful acnes. He was put on strong antibiotics that caused nose bleeds. When he stopped the meds and switched his hydration to only drinking H2 water, his severe acne cleared up in about 4-6 weeks. All of us are now super-healthy. As a family, we will always have an H2 water system for the rest of our lives!" – *Bill R. Holland Michigan*

Sleep, Energy, Digestion, High-Blood Pressure & High Cholesterol

As a hospital pharmacist for over 30 years, I expect science-based evidence to prove a therapy is effective. In 2011, I learned about ionized water and looked at some studies. I found mostly animal studies and anecdotal stories. Today, there are over 1,000 scientific studies! In just a few days of drinking and cooking with ionized, alkaline hydrogen water, I went from needing 9 hours of sleep to only 6. Every day, I wake up rested and full of energy. My workday is demanding and the extra energy improves my performance, especially now that I am nearly 60-years-old. My husband suffered from digestion issues (not being regular), high-blood pressure and high cholesterol. After several months on H2 water, no more laxatives, no more Statin meds and he regained energy and stamina. My husband is 64, but feels like he is in his 40s. – *Toban, Registered Pharmicist (R.Ph) & C.M.H.A., Pasadena California*

My Dog's Soft Tissue Injury & My Bursitis

I am a health nut. In 2018, I saw a newspaper ad that read: "Free Healthy Hydrogen H2 Learning." It also asked: "Should We All Be Drinking Hydrogen Water?" So, I attended a relaxed home water party that provided us with healthy food, H2 water and free gifts. The party was both fun and educational as we watched a fascinating video-slideshow on H2 water therapy. At the end, I knew Molly and I needed H2 water. At that time, I could not afford the system, so I bought some very high-quality, extra-thick dark amber glass half-gallon jugs and gallons of H2 water @ $4 a gallon from the couple who hosted the party. "Molly" is my precious 85-pound 11-year-old Lab/Boxer mix, whom I rescued when she was 18 months, and now suffers from a soft tissue injury on her left shoulder. In just 5 days of giving Molly hydrogen water, there was a bounce to her step with less limping. I eventually took Molly off her meds. I developed bursitis on my left knee a week before the party. My knee was all swollen and I could not bend or flex it without much pain. I refused to take anti-inflammatory/pain killer drugs. After just 2-3 weeks of drinking level 1 alkaline H2 water, I was able to bend and flex with no pain! About 4 weeks later, I bought my own hydrogen water system with 4 filters. As of this writing, my bursitis is gone! I am 77-years-old and plan for me & Molly to always drink H2 water and give it to any pets I may have in the future." – *Rosalind E., Rio Vista California*

Energy, Stamina, Hair Growing Back & Preventive Medicine

We bought our first ionizer in 2017. In the first few weeks of drinking H2 water at alkaline level 1, my wife started to feel more energetic and less sleepy. Now she drinks alkaline level 3 which has more molecular hydrogen and not only has she continued to have increased energy and stamina, she also noticed that areas of thinning hair are regenerating and growing back. My dear wife convinced me to try alkaline water and I now drink alkaline level 3 daily. As a surgeon who has been in practice for over 20 years, I need a lot of energy to give my patients the very best care possible. We consider our decision to buy a hydrogen water therapy system as 'preventive medicine' which is what I encourage my patients to practice." – *Dr. Yomi F. M.D., Colon and Rectal Surgeon, Frisco Texas*

"There's a new science called orthomolecular medicine. You correct chemical imbalance with amino acids, vitamins and minerals that are in the body." –
Margo Kidder, Actress, Activist & Health Enthusiast

Chapter Twenty-Three

Understanding Electrolytes

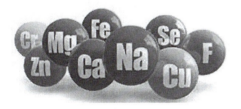

Electrolyte is a "medical/scientific" term for mineral salts, specifically ions. Electrolytes are sparks that keep our body running. They are necessary for life. They are what our cells (especially nerve, heart, muscle) use to maintain voltages across their cell membranes and to carry electrical impulses (nerve impulses, muscle contractions) across themselves and to our other cells. [1]

These electro-chemicals influence the body's pH — a chemical balance that determines how effectively our biological systems run. When there is a deficiency of body electricity, body functions slow down and eventually stop. Electrolytes are formed when certain minerals come together in solution and create electrical activity providing energy for our body. When electrolytes are dissolved, they break apart into charged particles called ions that create electricity.

Electrolytes facilitate delivery of oxygen to achieve and maintain peak brain function and proper nervous system response. The constant

---

[1] University of Waterloo, Canada website:
http://sciborg.uwaterloo.ca/~cchieh/cact/c120/electrolyte.html.

firing of micro-electric impulses across the synapses of our brain requires a great deal of energy. Only electrolytes can supply this. If, because of electrolyte imbalance, there is not enough oxygen available for nerve cells to fire when needed, our brain functions less effectively. Electrolytes help oxygen create a chemical reaction that allows our body to "burn" nutrients as fuel — which facilitates life!

Mineral & Electrolyte Supplementation

When our body is electrolyte deficient, vital nutrients are not oxidized enough. This compromises our ability to get fuel we need to run at peak performance and fight disease. Athletes know the value of electrolyte replacement after exercise. Electrolytes are a life-giving force lost in dehydration that can become a major health risk factor.

Approximately four percent of our body mass is composed of 21 macro and trace minerals that are essential for life. When mineral levels are insufficient to meet the demands of our body under emotional, physiological and psychological stresses such as during physical activity, the result will most likely be a substandard level of performance. For athletes or weekend exercisers, this increases the risk of serious injury and reduces the recovery rate after strenuous work or exercise. Most of us are not ingesting sufficient amounts of minerals because our food and water is mineral deficient. To compound problems, athletes often induce low body weights by maintaining restrictive diets which do not contain the variety of foods needed for ingesting a wide range of minerals. Certain foods or drinks can create mineral deficiency. For example, carbonated drinks containing high levels of phosphorus cause phosphorus to bind with calcium and move it out of our body. Calcium loss also increases following consumption of white sugar, salt or caffeine. Therefore, carbonated drinks used for rehydration should be avoided.

Did You Know Mineral Supplements Come in Different Sizes?

- Colloidal is the largest
- Chelated is smaller

- Ionic is smaller yet
- Ionic crystalloid dispersed in water becomes even smaller

Colloidal minerals are suspended in a liquid such as blood. They are too large to become dissolved. To get inside our cell membrane where minerals do their work, they must be dissolved in a solution. To be absorbed through our cell wall, a mineral must be smaller than the colloidal mineral form. Colloidal particles will readily pass through a filter paper, but they are too large to pass through a living membrane. [1] Colloidal particles cannot undergo osmosis. This means colloidal minerals are unable to get inside our cells. It may become debris floating around in our bloodstream looking for a nook or cranny to call home. These deposits may accumulate into arthritic conditions or kidney stones. Colloidal minerals were designed by nature to nourish plants after being broken down by organisms in the soil. Even plants won't use this large form of minerals unless they are munched up by critters in the dirt.

A plant can utilize minerals through chelation, which converts minerals into a form that is more assimilated by humans and animals. Ionic minerals are smaller than colloidal or chelated and have an even better chance of getting into our cells. When you put these ionic minerals into water they will break down into a solution known as **crystalloid**, which is highly absorbable. Minerals must get inside our cells to benefit our bodies. Water-dispersed forms of ionic minerals are assimilated 100 percent by our bodies, bypassing our digestive system, to provide electrical energy necessary to run our complex systems.

Are Higher Mineral Dosages Better?

Under most conditions, our body prefers minerals delivered in regular, bio-available smaller dosages. So, avoid mineral mega dosages! This is also true of trace minerals. They work in combination to provide a proper environment for electrolyte formation and maximum absorption. However, according Dr. G. Olarsch, N.D., too

---

[1] *Say No to Colloidal Minerals*, Sunset Adventures Press, Issue 4, June 1996.

few trace-minerals in a drink are unable to form a proper electrolyte balance to enter our cells and maximize rehydration. Only certain minerals will form electrolytes. For example, iron won't form electrolytes, but drinking electrolytes creates an electromagnetic energy in our body that will pull iron out from food and out of our blood into our cells. [1]

Key Minerals for Supplementation & Electrolyte Formation

Boron. A catalytic trace element that is suspected to play a role in prevention and treatment of osteoporosis as it aids in retention of calcium and magnesium in our bones. Studies indicate that boron improves the production of antibodies that help fight infection and decreases peak secretion of insulin from our pancreas. The way boron acts in our body is not fully understood. But a deficiency can cause abnormal bone formation.

Calcium. Most common mineral in our body. Adequate intakes of this mineral are an important determinant of bone health and risk of fracture. Calcium also carries an electric charge during an action potential across membranes and acts as an intracellular regulator and cofactor of enzymes and regulatory proteins. [2] Some research shows that a balance of 1:1 should be maintained with magnesium for homeostasis in the body. [3] The form of calcium supplementation should be specified. For example, calcium carbonate is common blackboard chalk and cannot be adequately absorbed by our body. A better choice would be calcium citrate or calcium aspartate. [4]

Chloride. As a natural salt of the mineral chlorine, chloride works with sodium and potassium to help us maintain healthy pH balance,

---

[1] Yarrow, David, *Fire in the Water*, Nature's Publishing, Ltd., 1999.
[2] Matkovic, Viliir, M.D., Ph.D., Connie Weaver, Ph.D., "Calcium," American Society for Nutritional Sciences, www.nutrition.org.
[3] Peiper, Howard, *Naturopathic Secrets for Building Better Bones*, Nature's Publishing Group, 2001.
[4] Martlew, Gillian, N.D., *Electrolytes the Spark of Life*, 1998 revised & updated, Nature's Publishing, Murdock FL.

nerve and muscle function. It also contributes to our digestion and waste elimination. Chloride should not be confused with the chemical chlorine used in water treatment. When chlorine is combined with waste in our digestive tract, there is a chemical reaction that produces trihalomethanes, a potential carcinogen. We can get plenty of chloride from a healthy diet of unprocessed foods.

Chromium. An essential nutrient required for healthy regulation of our blood sugar and fat metabolism. It protects against cardiovascular disease, diabetes, high cholesterol and can decrease body weight. Supplementation is needed if we eat white flour, milk and sugar as they steal chromium from our body and excrete it unused.

Cobalt. Helps absorb and process B_{12}, form red blood cells and treat anemia. It aids in repair of myelin, which surrounds and protects our nerve cells. Cobalt can also assist in our hormone production.

Copper. It works with our body's enzymes to help biochemical reactions occur in all cells. Copper is required for the absorption and utilization of iron and regeneration of blood. Copper and zinc together are crucial to the formation of collagen, connective tissues and the protein fibers found in our bone, cartilage, ligaments, dental tissues and skin. Deficiency symptoms are similar to iron deficiency and include anemia, cardiac abnormalities and elevated levels of serum cholesterol. Evidence exists that copper helps ease rheumatoid arthritis and other inflammatory diseases. Copper is utilized by most cells through enzymes involved in energy production, brain neurotransmitters and strengthening of our connective tissues.

Germanium. As a metallic trace mineral, it is known to improve cellular oxygenation. It also fights pain, assists in immune system operation, acts as an antioxidant and improves our stamina and endurance. Germanium acts as a carrier of oxygen to our cells.

Iodine. This is a nonmetallic element that is converted to iodide in our gut and absorbed through our digestive tract. Our thyroid gland needs this mineral to support metabolism, nerve and muscle function along with physical and mental development. Deficiencies can lead to reduced brain function, growth stunting, apathy, impaired movement, speech or hearing. Since soybeans, peanuts, cabbage, and turnips can block utilization of iodine, supplementation may be necessary for people who eat these foods.

Magnesium. This mineral facilitates 300 fundamental enzymatic reactions! It also functions in activation of amino acids and plays a key role in nerve transmissions and immune system operation. Numerous ATP-dependent reactions use magnesium as a cofactor.[1] This essential mineral enjoys a reciprocal relationship with calcium. In our muscles, calcium stimulates muscle fibers to tense up and contract whereas magnesium encourages our muscle fibers to loosen up and relax. Stored in the bones (60%) and muscles (40%), magnesium is called upon during exercise. Since bones do not release magnesium easily, muscles will give it up. The result may be cramps, irritability or twitching. Supplemental calcium and magnesium in a 1:1 ratio can be a healthy way to guard against this attack on our muscles.

Manganese. An element concentrated primarily in our bones, liver, pancreas and brain. Manganese factors into cholesterol metabolism, normal skeletal growth and development. Manganese is responsible for transmitting nerve impulses to our muscles along with RDA and DNA production. It is an important cofactor in the key enzymes of our glucose metabolism. Lack of manganese has also been implicated in aggravating bone loss and porosity.

Molybdenum. This is a component of many enzymes, including sulfite oxidase (deficiencies can cause disorders resulting in early age death). It is required for nitrogen metabolism. It is essential in working with vitamin B_2 in conversion of our food to energy and is necessary for iron utilization. Molybdenum deficiency is very rare but is linked to an increased allergic reaction to sulfite food additives (such as additives to wine).

---

[1] Berning, Jacqueline R., Nelson Steen, S., *Nutrition for sport and exercise,* Aspen Publishers, Gaithersburg, MD, 1998.

Potassium. Potassium performs countless vital functions supporting our nervous system, aiding in digestion and providing the electrolyte charge to our cells. Most of total body potassium is found in muscle tissue. Because of its link with metabolizing, oxygen-consuming parts of our body, a decline in total body potassium is usually interpreted as loss of muscle mass. This is not necessarily the case, but muscle mass loss is the result of a catabolic protein wasting condition which reduces total cell mass of the body. [1] Excess stress during exercise without proper nutrient components can facilitate this wasting condition. In some cases, low potassium can lead to death.

Phosphorus. As a key component of DNA, RNA, bones and teeth, phosphorus plays an important role in energy metabolism of our cells affecting carbohydrates, fatty acids, and proteins. It is essential for our bone formation and maintenance. It also stimulates muscle contraction. Deficiencies can appear as a general weakness, loss of appetite, bone pain and susceptibility to fractures. Excesses in the bloodstream may promote calcium loss.

Selenium. Shown to have a role in the detoxification of heavy metals, such as mercury, selenium plays a role in the production of antibodies in our immune system and may help prevent cancer and other degenerative diseases. Selenium protects our cell membranes, cell nuclei and chromosomes from environmental damage. Preliminary studies suggest that it may have an anti-cancer effect on humans. Toxic levels of selenium can cause hair loss, nail problems, accelerated tooth decay and swelling of our fingers.

Silicon. Plays a vital role in assisting calcium for growth, maintenance and flexibility of our joints and bones. Growing evidence suggests it may have anti-aging properties because it is a major player in preventing tissue degeneration and osteoporosis.

---

[1] Kehayias, Joseph J., Ph.D., Pierson, Richard N. Jr., M.D., American Society for Nutritional Sciences, 2001, www.nutrition.org.

Sodium. It works with potassium to maintain our body's proper water distribution and blood pressure. So, it is a primary mineral needed for our rehydration. It is also important to maintain our pH balance and facilitate transmission of our nerve impulses. People with pronounced losses of sodium through heavy perspiration or diarrhea may experience decreased blood volume and a fall in blood pressure that could result in shock. Excessive amounts of sodium can lead to cardiac failure and liver disease.

Zinc. Research reveals zinc is "a system within a system." It has its own absorption, homeostasis, bioavailability, excretion and feed-back loop mechanisms. [1] We need zinc to be healthy! It is vital to the function of 90 enzymes regulating dozens of bodily processes. It supports our immune system, fights infection, assists in chelating heavy metals, improves vision and sexual potency. Zinc aids in cell respiration, bone development, wound healing and regulation of heart rate and blood pressure. Zinc with copper is crucial to formation of connective tissues and protein fibers found in bone, cartilage, ligaments, dental tissues and skin. Zinc deficiency is a "malnutrition problem worldwide." So, zinc-rich foods should be included in our menus.

---

[1] https://www.ncbi.nlm.nih.gov/pmc/articles/PMC3724376/ J Res Med Sci 2013

"Nutrition is the only remedy that can bring full recovery and can be used with any treatment. Remember, food is our best medicine!" – Dr. Bernard Jensen

Chapter Twenty-Four

Adding Cellular Nutrition to H2 Water

Excessive production of free radicals caused by our polluted environment, stressful lifestyles and over-medicated society attack our bodies daily. Most of us are unable to fully defend this daily attack on our natural defense system.

Since the last century, nutritional medicine and supplementation has focused on replenishing nutritional deficiency. Countless hours and dollars have been spent to determine which nutrients our bodies have depleted. Blood tests, urine tests and hair samples have been conducted to determine which nutrients we need to supplement.

Mistakenly, we have been aiming at the wrong target. The present problem is not nutritional deficiency, but rather, underlying *oxidative stress*. Oxidative stress has been shown via medical research, to be the root cause of over 72 chronic degenerative diseases such as Heart Disease, Stroke, Cancer, Diabetes, Arthritis, Lupus, MS and more.

Because oxidative stress is our concern, we must determine what is a better approach to help prevent or control oxidative stress. This can be accomplished by bolstering our natural defenses through cellular nutrition delivered in H2 water.

Cellular nutrition is simply providing nutrients to our cells at optimum levels. This allows our cells to determine what they need. We do not have to worry which nutrients our cells are deficient in; we simply just provide the nutrients and our body does the rest.

Highly-respected Dr. Mark Smith, N.D., Ph.D, M.D. said: *"When it's really broken down, every single health issue, no matter the name, comes to cellular health."*

Cellular nutrition is providing our body with antioxidants along with supporting B vitamins and minerals at optimum levels. This is "preventative medicine" at its best because we can literally "attack" disease at its core by preventing oxidative stress from occurring.

Some may wonder if we can control oxidative stress by improving our diet and eating more fruits and vegetables. This is a good start. By eating 6 to 9 servings of organic fruits and vegetables each day, we can decrease the risk of heart attack, stroke, cancer, etc. Sadly, even if we maintain a great diet ... most of us can barely obtain the RDA level of all essential nutrients. Numerous medical studies have shown that less than 1% of the American population accomplishes this on a consistent basis.

One form of cellular nutrition that few have heard about are polysaccharides & polypeptides (PSP). They can provide a complete and balanced organic-based functional-food delivered to our cells via H2 water. PSP is a very potent, easy-to-digest whole food made from various strains of organic rice that can optimize our body's natural antioxidant, immune and repair systems. Oxidative stress can be controlled as our internal homeostasis is restored and protected.

Cellular nutrition is about health, not disease. Attacking the root cause of degenerative diseases is true preventative medicine. With PSP, we decrease our risk of developing degenerative diseases.

PSP and Hydrogen Water

A strong, healthy body depends on the condition of our cells, energy they produce and all internal systems achieving homeostasis. Therefore, it makes sense we keep our cells well-nourished.

This can easily be accomplished when we drink hydrogen water with PSP. Notice how PSP and H2 water complement each other.

- **Polysaccharides:** Biological fuel for cellular energy

- **Polypeptides:** Amino acids in the right quantities for our cells to perform their functions effectively and promote cellular renewal

- **Hydrogen Water:** H2 gas aids in delivery of food to sub-cellular levels. Keeps pH balanced in cells. Helps detoxify and give us electrolytes for cellular enzyme production.

Combining PSP with hydrogen water can slow down the cellular aging process, providing our body's cells with one of the highest essential nutrients to produce extra energy and assist in self-repair while increasing support of our cellular regeneration process.

Helpful Tips

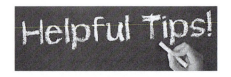

Before you continue to our Resource Directory, here are some tips that may help improve or even maximize your personal hydrogen water therapy experience:

H2 water is perfect for taking quality nutritional supplements. H2 aids in a more complete assimilation (absorption) of their nutrients.

Medication should be taken with the H2O non-ionized water. H2 may have a more potent effect. It has been recommended that medication be taken at least 30 minutes before or after drinking H2 water. You should work with a doctor or health practitioner when drinking H2 water. Some people have reduced or eliminated certain medications under a doctor's care, supervision and approval.

Drinking H2 water 20 minutes before every meal can help us distinguish between thirst and hunger. Many people do not eat as much. When H2 water is consumed before a meal, we also tend to chew more completely, rather than washing food down. It is also a good idea to drink another 8-16 ounces of H2 water 2-3 hours after each meal. In this way, H2 water is being consumed throughout the day.

Brewing coffee, tea or making any other acidic beverage with the higher alkaline (9-10 pH) H2 water can reduce acidity, improve taste and provide some H2 benefits.

Make ice cubes with higher alkaline (9-10 pH) H2 water can give same benefits as described above. Avoid plastic trays and only use food-grade 18/8 (18/304) stainless steel ice trays.

In **future editions**, we plan to have more Helpful Tips!

Resource Directory

Author's Recommendations

Water Ionizer Brands: The framework for Global Regulation & Oversight of Standards by International Associations is nearly complete. To meet those standards, we perform extensive research and testing to determine the highest-quality, most cutting-edge brand(s) that offer "best of the best" filtration medias and ionization design to produce consistent therapeutic doses of molecular hydrogen.

pHion Balance: A healthy well-balanced lifestyle company known for its easy-peezy urine & saliva pH test strips in convenient travel bottle. Committed to "greening our planet" by "greening" our bodies, their mission is to re-charge, re-energize and re-balance our lives. Read the pHion Balance "core values." Their cornerstone method is pH test strips that are practitioner-preferred, super-sensitive, precise, with a wide-range 4.5 to 9.0, and economical with 15-second results. Unconditional moneyback guarantee. Founded in 2002. BBB Accredited Business A+ Rating.

www.phionbalance.com   888-744-8589

AAA Water Ionizers: A wellness company and trusted source of research and accurate knowledge on H2 water therapy. AAA Water Ionizers offers one of the best hydrogen tablets, H2 Energize™, that meet the very strict BSCG "Gold Standard" for pro athletes. This formulation produces a consistent, therapeutic dose per tablet. With each bottle purchased, a donation is made to Molecular Hydrogen Institute to help fund more scientific research and clinical studies on H2 therapy.

www.aaawaterionizers.com   916-705-5001

Nutritional Resources

CELLULAR PSP - The polysaccharides and polypeptides in Cellular PSP (the original PSP) is a unique, organic-based functional food known to efficiently and effectively deliver a powerful combination of vital and essential nutrients to your body at the cellular level. Cellular PSP is from various strains of organic rice.

www.healthbesttoday.com

ACTIVIZE and MUNOGEN – Each have all-natural Non-GMO ingredients that are bioavailable to support energy-yielding metabolism and help increase blood flow throughout our bodies and brain. Available in 34 countries worldwide.

www.fitlineusa.us   312-752-7777

ELECTROBLAST™ – Pure electrolytes that support brain and body. ElectroBlast™ provides ionic multi trace-minerals dispersed in water (crystalloid) that contain more than just sodium and potassium found in some sports drinks.

www.electroblast.com

ZEOPOWDER – True form of the mineral zeolite that provides optimum benefits to aid elimination of heavy metals (arsenic, cadmium & mercury) and environmental toxins in a very gentle way.

www.zeohealth.com

VITAJUWEL – Their approach is based on age-old crystal healing traditions. They use a selection of hand-picked gems that are enclosed in glass bottles and vials. The gems' subtle vibration enhances drinking water.

www.VitaJuwel.com

Support & Inspiration

Center for the Arts – Rio Vista, Amanda Jenni: Non-profit. A place to pursue better health through creative work with equipment, supplies & instructors. Classes for kids & adults include fine arts, yoga, tai chi, movement, Zumba, dance and more. **www.centerfortheartsriovista.org** / **707-716-6136**

Peace in Body & Mind – Craig Petersen: Works with national & international philanthropic non-profits to rescue people from health crisis and restore balance in lives. Includes virtually eliminating polio worldwide & providing eye glasses for millions of children. **www.peaceinbodyandmind.org** / **707-430-5187**

Healthy Concepts of California – Fairfield, D.W. Chitwood, CMT: Dedicated to volunteer work. Essential oils advocate, National Holistic Institute Graduate, Certified Massage Therapist, health educator. **DwightChitwood@gmail.com** / **707-631-0409**

StopBottledWaterWaste - An organization working toward a planet free of plastic pollution and its toxic impact on all life. Dedicated to teaching communities how to replace plastic bottles with containers made from alternative materials that are both safe and easier to recycle. **www.stopbottledwaterwaste.com**

Institutions

Molecular Hydrogen Institute (MHI) collaborates with Universities and Institutions world-wide to advance all forms of H2 research, in part, to establish this NexGen discovery as a very safe medical gas therapy for diseases, athletics (athletes) or other conditions in terms of Prevention or Treatment.

MHI is the *epicenter of Hydrogen Education and Training*. We encourage all to visit the MHI website to learn more, get involved, take online courses for certification, attend conferences and support MHI by voluntary work or financial donations to accelerate this exciting Global Movement.

www.molecularhydrogeninstitute.org

H2 WATER 4 LIFE is a new entity established in 2018. Its mission is to research and bring accurate knowledge, initially by means of a new book, about H2 water therapy to a global audience. First edition is in English. However, we have agreements from volunteers to translate into more languages. We plan to become a non-profit and offer free H2 Learning Events throughout the world. All companies, individuals, charities, organizations, products or services that wish to work with **H2 WATER 4 LIFE** must compliment H2 water therapy & purpose of this book.

www.h2water4life.org

AAA Water Ionizers & H2 Research is a trusted source of scientific study and accurate knowledge on H2 water therapy along with NexGen water filter and ionizer technology. Free water quality reports, source water testing, consultations, presentations & classes are offered to small and large groups. Donations of time, ionizers & H2 therapy products to charities or those in need are reviewed on a case-by-case basis. Founders involved in water research and testing since 2005.

www.aaawaterH2research.org

At the Foot of Excellence®: A Ministry-Driven Volunteer Organization. Their mission is to bring physical, emotional and spiritual wellness to the community. At the core is providing free guide & service dogs for people living with visual impairments, physical disabilities and children with Autism Spectrum Disorder. A passion for helping neighbors achieve better health motivates many donations of time and technology. This ministry empowers each person to reach their own peak performance as they climb the mountain of life!

www.MiraDogsMission.com 418-325-1223

Bibliography

Anderson, N. and Peiper, H. "The Secrets of Staying Young", Safe Goods, Sheffield, MA 2008

Anderson, N. "Analyzing Sports Drinks", Safe Goods, Sheffield MA, 2002

Batmanghelidj, F. "Your Body's Many Cries for Water", Global Health Solutions, 1997

Bell, R. and Peiper, H. "The ADD & ADHD Diet", Safe Goods, Sheffield, MA2007

Clarke, Steven "What's In Your Water?" 2016-2018 (Rio Vista, California)

Clarke, Steven & Tina *"IN THE TRENCHES"* 2017-2018 (Rio Vista, California)

Diamond, J. and Cowden, W. "Cancer Diagnosis", Alternative Medicine, 2000

Emoto, M. "The True Power of Water", Beyond Words, 2005

Ingram, C. "The Drinking Water Book", Celestial Arts, 2006

Jhon, M. S. "The Water Puzzle and the Hexagonal Key", Uplifting Press, 2004

Peiper, H. "The Best in Natural Pet Care", Walk the Talk Productions, 2014

Sierra, Claudine. Consultant at University for International Cooperation, Principal Researcher in a TNC Program & audit for Rainforest Alliance and Ecological Flag, Costa Rica. "Earth Survey" & "Environmental Survey" 2006

Tunsky, G. "The Battle for Health is over pH", Crusador Enterprises, 2007

About the Authors

Dr. Howard Peiper is a Doctor of Naturopathic Medicine. In 1972, he received his degree in Naturopathy. After a decade in private practice, Dr. Peiper focused on Holistic Healing and became a successful consultant, speaker and writer.

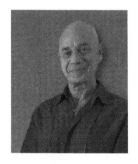

Over the years, his cutting-edge articles appeared in numerous medical journals and magazines. He also serves on the medical advisory board for several nutritional companies.

Dr. Peiper has written several bestselling titles, including: *The A.D.D. and A.D.H.D. Diet, The Secrets to Staying Young* and *New Hope for Serious Diseases.* He is a frequent guest speaker on radio and television programs. He even hosted his own shows, including the award-winning television show, "Partners in Healing."

Steven began his alternative, naturopathic journey in 1988 when he discovered Dr. Bernard Jensen. Steven bought nearly all of his books. From that foundation, he rapidly studied nutrition and many forms of alternative naturopathic health care.

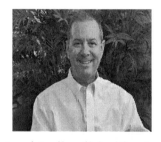

A life-changed injury in 2004 exposed Steven to virtually all legitimate forms of holistic healing. In 2005, he experienced his "Ah-Ha" moment at a Texas health conference on water where, by chance, Dr. Paul Yanick was a guest speaker. Later, Dr. Yanick diagnosed a deadly infection, rushed Steven into surgery and saved his life. Since that near-death experience, Steven has devoted a big part of his life to studying the truth and science of water. This study led to crossing paths with MHI and Howard. Today, Steven is a respected Certified Molecular Hydrogen Advisor, Nano Hydration Specialist, researcher consultant, instructor, nutritionist and writer. Currently, he trains others via a webinar program live-streamed throughout North America, *"IN THE TRENCHES"* and writes a newspaper column, "What's In Your Water?"

Printed in Poland
by Amazon Fulfillment
Poland Sp. z o.o., Wrocław